CW00363248

ESSENTIALS FOR MEN

health&
fitness

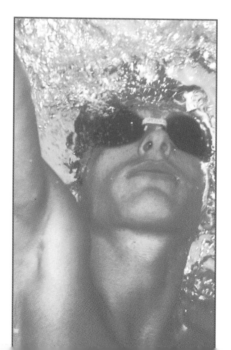

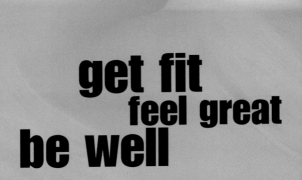

get fit
feel great
be well

ESSENTIALS FOR MEN

health&
fitness

alex smith

ESSENTIALS FOR MEN: HEALTH & FITNESS
Alex Smith

First published in 2000 by Mitchell Beazley,
an imprint of Octopus Publishing Group Ltd
2–4 Heron Quays, London El4 4JP
Copyright © Octopus Publishing Group Ltd 2000

Executive Editor	**Rachael Stock**
	Vivien Antwi
Executive Art Editor	**Kenny Grant**
Project Editor	**Jane Cooke**
	Michelle Bernard
Art Editor	**Christine Keilty**
Design	**Lovelock & Co**
Production	**Nancy Roberts**
Picture Research	**Jenny Faithfull**
	Lois Charlton
Index	**Hilary Bird**
Illustrations	**Jim Robbins**
	Halli Verrinder
Special Photography	**Steve Gorton**
Medical Consultant	**Dr Abi Berger, MRCGP**

ISBN 1-84000-319-7

A CIP catalogue record for this book is available from
the British Library.

Front cover: Image Bank

Typeset in Baskerville, Flyer, Impact and Syntax

Printed in China by Toppan Printing Company Ltd

Contents

Introduction

It's no coincidence that men in developed countries have the highest incidence of cancer and heart disease in the world. Two of the prime causes of these diseases are bad diet and lack of exercise and modern corporate life contributes to both.

Healthy is fun

Being desk-bound eight hours a day means that many of us don't get the exercise our bodies require. For some men any break at work is more likely to be for a cigarette than exercise. Twenty-first century living doesn't encourage healthy eating either. Many men are too busy trying to combine their family, work, and social lives to think about the food they eat. Food gets chosen because it's convenient rather than healthy. It doesn't have to be this way. There are many ways of improving your health and fitness that aren't lifestyle threatening. Cooking up recipes using delicious fresh ingredients, playing five-a-side football with your mates, and having regular sex all help you to stay in shape. Nobody ever said that staying healthy couldn't be fun.

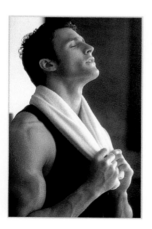

Warning Signs

However healthy our lifestyles we are still prone to illness from time to time. How quickly we recover depends on our ability to recognise the body's warning signs. Unfortunately, men are notorious for ignoring symptoms of illness. This 'head in the sand' approach means that diseases are often fairly advanced before they are diagnosed by doctors, which makes a full recovery less likely. Some of the symptoms of the most serious diseases are impossible to detect without the help of your GP. Regular medical check-ups ensure that illness can be diagnosed early and treated quickly.

Eating fit

Food provides the carbohydrates, protein, fat, vitamins, minerals, water, and fibre our bodies need to function properly. Knowing the effects they have on the body can help you make an informed choice about your diet. The common mistake many men make is to eat too much food containing fat, such as red meat, and not enough containing carbohydrates, vitamins, and fibre, such as vegetables and fruit. Most men could also benefit from drinking a lot less alcohol and more water.

Downing too much booze not only leads to painful hangovers, it also increases the risk of heart disease, liver disease, and ulcers and can trigger depression and violent behaviour. And, like smoking, it can lead to impotence.

Health check

There's a feeling of great relief when recovering from illness but it would be better if the medical problem hadn't arisen in the first place. You can reduce your risks of being ill by taking preventative measures such as doing regular exercise and steering clear of cigarettes. There's good news for moderate drinkers here, as it's been found that those who drink a glass or two of alcohol every day (but no more) are less susceptible to heart disease.

Stress

Stress is an underlying factor behind many diseases and this can easily build up without you realising it. Reducing your workload, making more spare time for yourself, mentally leaving behind your work when you go home, and improving relationships with your friends and family all help to smooth furrowed brows.

Major diseases

The chances are you'll never suffer from a serious illness, but it's important to know about them so you can recognise the symptoms and take action to avoid them. With today's medicine, serious diseases such as cancer don't necessarily mean the beginning of the end. If the disease is detected early enough and treated correctly there's no reason why you can't make a full recovery and continue to lead a long and active life.

Major causes of death

1 Heart attack
2 Stroke
3 Cancer of the lung, trachea, and bronchial tubes
4 Emphysema, chronic bronchitis, and other lung problems
5 Pneumonia
6 Traffic accidents
7 Suicide
8 Stomach cancer
9 Colon and rectal cancer
10 Cirrhosis of the liver

Ranging from heart attacks to cirrhosis of the liver, all have one thing in common: they are all less likely to occur in men who look after themselves. Which means those who eat sensibly, exercise, avoid stress, drink alcohol in moderation, and don't smoke stand a very good chance of defying these killers.

Waiting list

Men have a problem with doctors. They regard a visit to the GP as a sign of weakness and they are too proud to relinquish control over their bodies to others. There is no merit in stoically enduring an illness. Doctors don't just cure you of ailments, they also help to keep you healthy in the first place by way of preventative medicine. For this to be effective your doctor should be somebody whom you can trust and talk to. If you can't discuss your problems openly, your GP won't know how you're feeling and it will be difficult to diagnose your complaints. Embarrassment over discussing sexual matters could have serious consequences, because sexual functioning is a barometer of general health. Getting used to going to the doctor regularly will help with this and also prevent a build-up of fear of the unknown.

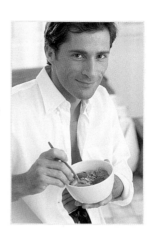

Regular help from medical professionals will also help you deal with problems as you age.

Toning up

Everybody benefits from exercise and you're never too old or unfit to build up your strength, flexibility, and aerobic fitness. Working out or playing sports builds muscles, reduces fat, improves cardiovascular fitness, and de-stresses the body.

All these things make you less prone to heart disease, certain cancers, and a wide range of other disorders. Exercise will also boost your sexual performance and improve your immune system. You will feel fitter, look good, and be better equipped to face life's challenges. Any exercise programme should take into account your fitness, age, and lifestyle. Finding the right programme for you is easier if you speak to a personal trainer or gym staff member.

Exercises

Full body exercises such as squats; heel raises; dumbbell flies, rows, and raises; triceps presses; crunches; toe reaches; and leg, hip, groin, back, side, chest, and pectoral stretches all help strengthen muscles and increase flexibility. When doing any exercise, be careful not to overstretch the muscles. Use slow, controlled movements until you feel a slight tug in the muscle. Then you know it's time to stop. Don't risk an injury.

The right diet

Eating for life

Busy lives often mean that men leave their diets to chance. By learning the basics of good nutrition you should be able to enjoy good health – whether you're working late at the office or training for a marathon.

The right food

• Food provides the nutrients your body needs for survival and good health. There are six main nutrient groups – proteins, carbohydrates, fats, vitamins, minerals, and water. Fibre isn't a nutrient, but it is a very important part of a healthy diet.

• Each man's dietary requirements are unique and factors, such as lifestyle, body type, and genes, all determine nutritional needs. However, there are broad rules that should form the basis of all diets: eat plenty of fruit, vegetables, and grains; drink lots of water; and minimise your fat intake.

• The food pyramid (see p.20) tells you what foods to place at the heart of your diet, what to eat in moderation, and what to leave on the supermarket shelf. This is the starting point if you're going to take control of your eating habits.

• If you follow the food pyramid logic, chances are you'll have to part company with some old friends. Fatty and sugary foods will increase both your girth and your chances of getting heart disease, so prepare to ditch some of the following: meat, especially beef and pork products, dairy products, mayonnaise, biscuits, cakes, and doughnuts. If you have high cholesterol levels, it's particularly important to avoid too much saturated fat – found in animal products, including meat and eggs.

• Once you understand your nutritional requirements, you need to devise a game plan. Start by writing down the changes you want to make ("I want to eat less sugar and more complex carbohydrates"). Say why you want to make these changes ("Cut the risk of heart disease"), and write down achievable goals ("Eat fish instead of steak twice a week").

Nourishing facts

• Proteins help in the body's growth and repair of cells, muscles, and skin.
• Carbohydrates are burned for energy and keep skin, bones, and nails healthy.
• Fats are burned and also stored for future energy needs. They also insulate against heat loss.
• Vitamins regulate metabolism and are vital for growth, digestion, and reproduction.
• Minerals are inorganic substances that are involved in countless chemical processes.
• Water cools and lubricates the body and transports nutrients through the circulatory system. It flushes out waste and toxins.
• Fibre keeps the digestive tract clean and functioning well.

Common eating mistakes

• **Skipping breakfast** Start the day with a decent-sized breakfast consisting of cereal, skimmed milk, and fruit juice rather than artery-clogging bacon, egg, and sausages.
• **Eating too much fat** Saturated fat converts into cholesterol, which puts extra pressure on the heart.
• **Crash dieting** Quick-fix diets don't work in the long term.
• **Eating irregularly** Fasting for four to six hours or more lowers your blood sugar levels, leading to irritability and fatigue.
• **Drinking too much alcohol** Limit your consumption. More than three units a day can lead to addiction, illness, or accidents.

Instant ways to eat well

• **Take more fibre** It reduces cholesterol, protects you from colon cancer, and helps prevent irregular bowel function.
• **Snack away** Healthy snacking can help boost energy levels, but steer clear of chocolates and sweets. Instead go for fruit, wholemeal bread, and vegetable sticks.
• **Sleep empty** Don't eat just before bedtime as it's likely to cause insomnia, indigestion, or heartburn. Have only a light meal for supper and eat the day's main meal at lunchtime.
• **Go low-fat** Look for low-fat alternatives of your fatty favourites. If you eat beef or pork, for example, go for the leanest cuts available.

Major food groups

1 **Proteins** These complex molecules make up 15–20 percent of your body weight and provide the body's main building materials. When you digest food, your body turns the large protein molecules (from poultry, fish, and eggs, for example) into amino acids. These smaller molecules are then put back together again to form the main ingredients for the growth and repair of skin, bones, muscles, hair, teeth, and all other types of body tissue. Note that a high protein intake, perhaps including supplements, doesn't necessarily turn you into a muscleman. It does, however, provide the raw material if you are exercising at sufficiently high levels to build up muscle.

2 **Carbohydrates** These are found in sugars (refined sugar, honey, and treacle) and starches (vegetables, fruit, pulses, and whole grains). They are burned by the body at varying speeds to generate the energy needed for us to grow, repair ourselves, move around, and keep warm. Sugars are known as simple carbohydrates, because they are quickly digested into glucose (blood sugar), which is metabolised into energy by our muscles and organs. Starches are complex carbohydrates and are broken down into glucose and absorbed into our bloodstreams in a slower and more controlled manner. As well as providing energy, carbohydrates have other vital roles. They help to break up the fat that can lead to obesity and heart disease, and they contribute to the appearance and health of skin, bones, and nails.

3 **Fats** Yes, as we all should know by now, too much fat-laden food can lead to increased waistlines and clogged arteries, but fat is still a vital component of your diet. It's burned as energy and stored for future use in case other energy sources run low. Fat teams up with proteins to form membranes (semi-permeable skins) around every cell. Fat also insulates the body from heat loss as it is laid down in layers beneath the skin. It cushions vital organs, such as the kidneys and liver, by growing in "pads" around them.

Where to find them

1 **Proteins** Fish, seafood, poultry, lean
meat, and offal are all rich sources
of proteins, since they are made
from animal cells. Eggs and dairy
products also contain proteins
because in nature they are the
natural products providing nourishment
for the growth of animals.
Plant seeds Beans, whole grains, maize, and nuts are all rich
in proteins, in addition to containing large amounts of
complex carbohydrates. These foodstuffs are particularly
important to vegetarians and vegans, as they will form their
only source of protein. Between 50–110g (2–4oz) of protein
foods should be consumed daily.

2 **Complex carbohydrates** These are generally found in the
fleshy parts of vegetables, fruits, pulses, and grains. Foods,
such as bread, pasta, rice, kidney beans, and avocados, all
contain high levels of complex carbohydrates. They tend to
be heavy and filling foods, and should make up to two-
thirds of your daily food intake.
Simple carbohydrates These are characterised by their
sweetness. Treacle, syrup, honey, and confectionery are all
high in simple carbohydrates, and refined sugar is a pure
source. They are good for instant energy, but should make
up only a small fraction of your daily intake. They contain
little nutritional value and also contribute to tooth decay.

3 **Fats** All fats derived from animal sources are saturated.
Although the body will readily digest them, their intake
should be kept to a minimum, because of the detrimental
effects they can have if they start building up in the body.
Palm and coconut oils are also saturated.
Unsaturated oils are far more beneficial in the diet.
Vegetable oils are polyunsaturated (partly saturated), while
olive oil is monounsaturated. Olive oil is the most beneficial
to the body. Because of the high levels of carbohydrates
needed in your diet, fats and oils should only represent some
5 percent of your daily intake. Many men consume far in
excess of this percentage.

Vital vitamins

Vitamins are only needed in relatively small quantities, but without them we begin to malfunction. Most vitamins cannot be produced by our bodies, so it's crucial that we include them in a healthy diet that includes a wide variety of different foods.

Vitamin check list

WATER SOLUBLE VITAMINS

• **Vitamin C** is an antioxidant necessary for building bones, forming neurotransmitters, which transmit electrical signals, and detoxifying the liver. It boosts immunity and helps prevent colds. **Good sources:** Oranges, grapefruit, red peppers, raw spinach, potatoes, broccoli, Brussels sprouts. **Daily requirement:** 60mg

• **Thiamin (Vitamin B_1)** helps convert carbohydrates to energy. Deficiency may cause fatigue and appetite loss. **Good sources:** Peas, beans, whole grains, pork. **Daily requirement:** 1.4mg

• **Riboflavin (Vitamin B_2)** helps create energy from food. Vital in the formation of red blood cells and hormones. Helps maintain tissues. **Good sources:** Milk products, whole grains, broccoli, asparagus, potatoes, oranges, eggs, liver. **Daily requirement:** 1.6mg

• **Niacin (Vitamin B_3)** helps create energy from food. **Good sources:** Grains, cereals, baked foods, meat, poultry, fish, peanuts, beer. **Daily requirement:** 18mg

• **Pantothenic acid (Vitamin B_5)** helps metabolise food and helps produce key hormones and neurotransmitters. **Good sources:** All animal and vegetable tissue. **Daily requirement:** 6mg

• **Vitamin B_6** helps regulate the nervous system. Important in breaking down protein and amino acids and converting them into energy. Also helps in the metabolism of glucose and fatty acids, and in the production of red blood cells. **Good sources:** Whole grains, potatoes, chicken, fish, egg yolks, bananas, avocados. **Daily requirement:** 2mg

• **Vitamin B$_{12}$** is essential for DNA synthesis, and cell production and division. **Good sources:** Liver, oysters, beef, pork, whole-milk dairy products, eggs. **Daily requirement:** 1mcg (microgram)

• **Folic acid** is required for the growth and division of cells and the formation of haemoglobin. **Good sources:** Beans, cereals, spinach, asparagus, broccoli, okra, various seeds, liver. **Daily requirement:** 200mcg

• **Biotin** helps immune system function. Vital in food metabolism and the formation of proteins, hormones, and neurotransmitters. **Good sources:** Peanut butter, pulses, nuts, grains, egg yolks, offal, yeast, cauliflower. **Daily requirement:** 0.15mcg

FAT SOLUBLE VITAMINS
• **Vitamin A** is required for normal vision, reproduction, cell development, growth, and immunity. It maintains the health of the skin and membranes. Beta-carotene, which converts to vitamin A in the body, is an antioxidant (*see p.75*). **Good sources:** Peaches, carrots, spinach, broccoli, tomatoes, lettuce, green beans, fish, liver, egg yolks, whole milk. **Daily requirement:** 800mcg

• **Vitamin D** is key to bone building, healthy teeth, and nerve-muscle interaction. **Good sources:** Sunshine, canned sardines, salmon, fortified dairy products. **Daily requirement:** 5mcg

• **Vitamin E** is an antioxidant. It lowers cholesterol and helps prevent a build up of plaque in arteries. It boosts immunity, helps prevent cataracts, and may help prevent heart disease. **Good sources:** Nuts, sunflower seeds, green leafy vegetables, wheat germ, whole grains. **Daily requirement:** 100mg

• **Vitamin K** helps regulate blood clotting. **Good sources:** Green, leafy vegetables, fruit, seeds, eggs, dairy products, meat. **Daily requirement:** 60–80mcg

Must-have minerals

Minerals are not as specifically linked to particular foods as vitamins, so a less varied diet will usually provide them. You must aim for maximum variety, however, for the sake of your vitamin needs. The minerals listed below are the ones you need the most of.

Mineral check list

1 **Calcium** is key to building bones and teeth among other important roles. It may protect against high blood pressure and colon cancer. Good sources: Dairy products, sardines, broccoli, leafy vegetables. Daily requirement: 800mg

2 **Chloride** is another essential mineral, primarily for the nervous system and for maintaining fluid balance. Good sources: Table salt. Daily requirement: 300–400mg

3 **Magnesium** is a bone-builder that helps regulate the heart and protects against heart disease. Important in enzyme activity, and in metabolism. Good sources: Green leafy vegetables, pulses, seafood, nuts, soya beans, eggs, whole grains, dairy products. Daily requirement: 300mg

4 **Phosphorus** is vital for bone building, it helps maintain the body's fluid balance, and is important in metabolism. Good sources: Dairy products, meat, fish, grains, nuts, beans. Daily requirement: 800mg

5 **Potassium** regulates blood pressure and heart function. It's vital for muscle contraction and transmission of nerve impulses. Good sources: Citrus fruits, bananas, most other fruits and vegetables, seafood. Daily requirement: 3500mg

6 **Sodium** is also important in the transmission of nerve impulses, regulating blood pressure, and in metabolism. Good sources: Natural foods; added to many canned and frozen foods, cereals, and crisps. Daily requirement: 2400mg

Other diet essentials
Water – why we need it

• Water really is the elixir of life, for without it nothing could live. It serves many purposes in your body: it's a medium for carrying substances around the body; it provides the lubrication for your movements; and it holds your cells rigid.

• Good old H_2O absorbs the goodness from your digested food and carries waste away in your urine. It enables you to shed tears and allows you to sweat. Water accounts for around 80 percent of your body mass, and you will die if you allow yourself to dehydrate by only a few percent.

• Water is obtained from drinks and food. It may seem unnecessary to remind someone to consume enough water, but some people do not register a thirst when they are dehydrating. It's also worth remembering that extreme perspiration, crying, and a runny nose can all lead to both dehydration and extreme cramps from the loss of salt in sweat, tears, and mucus. Heavy consumption of alcohol has a similar effect.

Fibre facts

• Fibre is not absorbed into the body at all. Nevertheless, it's vital for good health – helping you digest and preventing constipation.
• It's the material in plant food (vegetables, fruit, grains) that your body can't digest.
• Fibre gives a full feeling without the extra calories.
• It cleans the digestive tract as it passes along it.
• The recommended daily intake is 20–30g ($^3/_4$ –1oz).

Sources of fibre

All-bran cereal (85g [3oz])	8.6g
Apple (with skin)	2.8g
Brussels sprouts (180g [6oz])	5.0g
Bread slice (wholemeal)	2.4g
Green peas (100g [4oz])	5.4g
Kidney beans (85g [3oz])	6.9g
Lentils (85g [3oz])	5.2g
Orange (small)	2.9g
Potato (medium, baked)	5.0g
Spaghetti (140g [5oz], wholemeal)	5.4g

The food pyramid

Use the pyramid to check if you're consuming a variety of foods in the right proportions. Eat plenty of foods from the lower two tiers, but consume those near the top sparingly.

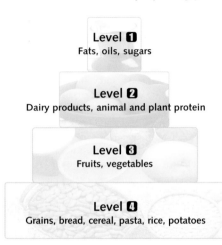

Level 1
Fats, oils, sugars

Level 2
Dairy products, animal and plant protein

Level 3
Fruits, vegetables

Level 4
Grains, bread, cereal, pasta, rice, potatoes

Level 1
Fats, oils, sugars, sweets, and confectionery: 1/2–1 1/2 daily servings. One serving = four teaspoons of sugar or oil, or two chocolate bars

Level 2
Dairy products and proteins: 4–6 daily servings. One serving = a mug of milk, 25g (1oz) hard cheese, 90g (3½oz) lean meat

Level 3
Fruits: 2–4 servings. One serving = a piece of fruit, or a half mug of fruit juice. Vegetables: 3–5 servings. One serving = a handful of raw vegetables, or a half mug of juice

Level 4
Grains, bread, cereal, pasta, rice, potatoes: 6–11 servings. One serving = medium bread slice, or half bowl of cereal

Your own food processor

What happens to food after you eat? Before your body can use the food, it must be broken down and converted into substances in the digestive tract that your body can use.

STAGE **1** THE MOUTH

The thought of food will already have triggered the release of saliva and mucus in your mouth. Your teeth and tongue cut, mash, and mix the food, while chemicals in saliva help break it down before it's swallowed in small amounts.

STAGE **2** THE STOMACH

Hydrochloric acid and other gastric juices attack the food, and powerful muscle contractions churn it until it becomes a soupy liquid called chyme.

STAGE **3** THE SMALL INTESTINE

The liquid drains into the small intestine where it's met by enzymes secreted by the liver, pancreas, and gallbladder that finish digestion. This long intestine is coated with millions of hair-like structures called villi through which the food (now refined chemicals) is absorbed. These chemicals will travel to every cell in the body via the bloodstream and the highways of the lymph system.

STAGE **4** THE LARGE INTESTINE

Excess water and remaining useful minerals are absorbed back into the body through the large intestinal (or colon) wall. What is left passes into the rectum as faeces and leaves the body through the anus after several hours.

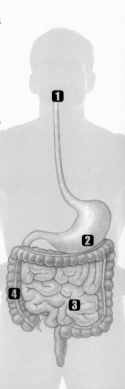

Weighty matters

Not only is obesity a turn-off, it also has serious consequences for your health. Many of us are overweight today due to sedentary lifestyles and high-fat diets, but attaining a healthy weight is the greatest asset to health.

Are you overweight?

If you are more than 20 percent above your optimal body weight or wearing 25 percent body fat, you're at risk. Check how much you should weigh using the chart opposite.

Why does it matter?

If you fall within the danger zones it means you're more susceptible to high blood pressure, clogged arteries, strokes, heart attacks, and colon and prostate cancer.

Putting weight on

If you're over 30, healthy, and your weight is increasing at a steady pace, don't worry. At this age a man's metabolic rate starts to slow down, which often leads to an average weight gain of 500–700g (18–25oz) a year.

What is cholesterol?

Cholesterol is a soft, fat-like substance, which the liver uses to help form cell membranes (semi-permeable skins) and hormones (chemical messengers). Cholesterol is produced by the liver and much of it comes from our food. If you consume too many foods rich in saturated fats you'll have more cholesterol than your body needs. Excess cholesterol clings to artery walls as fatty deposits, which can eventually cause blockages. Such obstructions can, in turn, lead to heart attacks and strokes. If you have a history of heart disease or high cholesterol in your family, get a cholesterol check at your doctor's surgery.

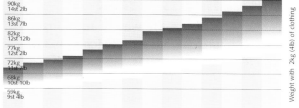
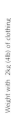

Weight with 2kg (4lb) of clothing

1.60m 1.62m 1.65m 1.67m 1.70m 1.72m 1.75m 1.78m 1.80m 1.82m 1.85m 1.87m 1.90m 1.93m
5' 3" 5' 4" 5' 5" 5' 6" 5' 7" 5' 8" 5' 9" 5' 10" 5' 11" 6' 0" 6' 1" 6' 2" 6' 3" 6' 4"

Height wearing 2.5cm (1in) heels

Large build
Medium build
Small build

Top three causes of weight gain

1 **Eating too much** Most of us eat more food than our bodies actually need. If you eat more calories than you burn, the excess gets converted into fat, which is stored in fat cells.

2 **Lack of exercise** If you want to burn off excess calories and avoid getting fat, you need to exercise. Get off your butt if you want to lengthen your lifespan.

3 **Fat genes** It's not entirely your parents' fault, but you are genetically programmed to carry a certain amount of fat. It's no excuse for lack of exercise though.

Draw a line from your weight on the left to your waist size on the right. The point where the line intersects the central scale will give you an estimate of your body fat percentage.

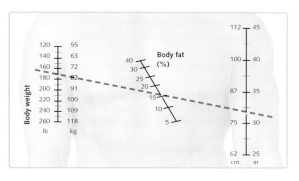

Shedding the flab

Eating fat is a sure-fire way of acquiring a fuller figure. Fat has over twice as many calories as carbohydrates and proteins, and it isn't converted into energy as quickly. So the simple message is...

Eat less fat

Cutting fat from your diet is the key to weight loss. Experts say that you should get only five percent of calories from fat, and if you want to lose weight you should be aiming for even less than this. Eat more complex carbohydrates, such as vegetables, fruit, wholemeal bread, and pulses. Not only do they provide lots of minerals and vitamins, but they are also fat burners as your body has to work harder to digest them.

Do more exercise

Just cutting back on fat will not make you lose weight. Exercise is missing from the equation. Aerobic exercise (sustained, rhythmic exercise using large body muscles) steps up the rate at which your body burns fuel. Try 30 minutes of jogging, cycling, swimming, football, or tennis three times a week.

Cutting cholesterol

To lower your cholesterol levels limit your intake of saturated fat. Foods to avoid include red meat, pork, dairy products made from whole milk (cheese, butter, yogurt, ice cream, sour cream), coconut oil, and fried foods. The pure cholesterol content of what you eat is not as crucial in raising blood cholesterol as the levels of saturated fat. But to be on the safe side, go easy on high-cholesterol foods, such as eggs and shrimps. Those people that are genetically predisposed towards high cholesterol levels (if it runs in the family) should be very strict about sticking to such guidelines.

Top ten tips for fat fighting

1 **Slash and burn** The only way to melt excess blubber in the long term is to burn more calories than you consume. That's why you need long-term strategies, such as cycling instead of driving to work, and switching to low-fat milk.

2 **Crash diets** Crash diets don't work even if you can bear the regimes. Your metabolism slows down when you stop eating and takes a while to return to normal when you start again.

3 **Fat substitutes** Learn to live without high-fat favourites by substituting them with tasty alternatives. Sorbet instead of ice cream, for instance, or dried apricots instead of peanuts.

4 **Don't torture yourself** If you push too hard to curtail fat, you'll just get frustrated and switch back. It's still OK to eat ice cream – just not every day.

5 **Packed lunches** If the canteen's lunchtime special is stodge and chips, why not take in your own low-fat lunch? Maybe pack a lean chicken sandwich and always include fruit.

6 **Night pickings** Your digestive capacity drops by 20 to 40 percent at night, and when you go to bed you're not exercising to burn it off (well, not all night).

7 **Savour the flavour** It takes about 20 minutes for your body's feedback system to realise you've had enough food. If you eat too quickly you'll unwittingly eat more that you need.

8 **Read the labels** The nutritional information panels on food packets give details about fat and calorie contents. Use them to make informed choices about what you eat.

9 **Cut back on booze** If you're trying to lose weight, cut out booze. Alcoholic drinks contain calories with little nutritional value but plenty of potential to expand your waistline.

10 **Lighten the dessert** When you're craving something sweet after your main course go for something light and non-fatty, like a nice, crunchy apple which has no fat and few calories.

Drinking to your health

All hail to the ale and a cheer for the beer!
Yes, alcohol is great, but only if you drink a
sensible amount. Science tells us that moderate
drinkers have healthier hearts and live longer
than heavy drinkers and teetotallers.

Booze benefits

Not only does moderate drinking help you relax and give you
a mild sense of euphoria, it can also help to prevent heart
attacks and strokes. Alcohol increases your levels of HDL
cholesterol, which helps carry away the artery-clogging LDL
cholesterol. It also decreases the blood's ability to form clots.

And the bad news...

Medical research has shown that if you cross the line from
moderate drinking all the positive effects go down the tube.
Instead of preventing heart disease, drinking can actually
cause it by raising the risk of heart attacks and strokes by
damaging heart muscles and raising blood pressure.

Heavy drinking problems

• Drinking too much alcohol has implications for every organ
in your body. Brain cells are destroyed, nerve damage can lead
to impotence, and toxins damage sperm. Liver cancer or
cirrhosis may develop, and digestion is impaired. Alcohol
abuse also gives rise to a range of social problems. Half of all
traffic deaths, for example, and at least a quarter of murders
and suicides are alcohol-related.
• The effects of drinking differ widely between individuals,
but at some point the ill effects of too much drink will concern
everybody. While moderate drinkers experience feelings of
relaxation, exhilaration, and increased sexual desire, heavier
drinkers may experience hangovers, disrupted sleep, slurred
speech, memory lapses, impaired judgement, and depression
– as well as the health problems listed above.

Top five hangover cures

While we may not realise the long-term damage drinking too much alcohol does to our bodies, we all know what the short-term consequence is – the dreaded hangover. You might not be able to eliminate nausea, dizziness, and a pounding headache, but you'll be able to make the morning after more bearable if you follow these tips:

1 **Fruit juice** A glass of orange juice will help speed the removal of any remaining alcohol in your bloodstream.

2 **Pain relief** To alleviate headaches take a mild pain reliever, such as paracetamol or aspirin.

3 **Drink water** Two or three glasses of plain water will hinder dehydration – one of the causes of a hangover. Try to drink two to three glasses before you go to bed.

4 **Vitamin C** Take a supplement, or eat fruit that's rich in vitamin C, such as oranges, grapefruit, and strawberries.

5 **Be patient** The only thing that really heals a hangover is time. In about 24 hours you'll feel a lot better.

Safe limits

The benefits of alcohol depend on moderation. For most men that means no more than three units of alcohol a day. (A unit is defined as a half pint of beer or one glass of wine). The limit for men endorsed by the British Medical Association is 21 units a week, but many men drink more than this. There are other ways you can make drinking safer as well as unit watching. Eat something first as food in the stomach slows absorption and reduces the severity of hangovers. Drink more slowly – try and make one drink last an hour. Don't drink every day otherwise you'll build up a tolerance and drink more. Alternate alcoholic with non-alcoholic drinks and leave the bubbly for special occasions because fizzy drinks are absorbed faster into the bloodstream.

Complete health guide

Self health check
You and your doctor
Fighting fatigue
Headaches
Dizziness and fainting
Anxiety
Depression
Fever
Skin problems
Coughs and sore throats
Sneezes
Sore throats
Breathing problems
Abdominal problems
Nausea and vomiting
Bowel problems
Muscle soreness
Joint problems
Back pain
Sports injuries

Self health check

None of us are saints and from time to time we all put our health on the line. But while the occasional bout of hedonism is OK, be wary of falling into too many bad habits.

Good habits

• Base your eating around energy-giving foods, like pasta, bread, and rice and eat plenty of fruit and vegetables.
• Drink lots of water to prevent dehydration. Keep a big bottle of mineral water near you every day.
• Spend 30 minutes three times a week doing aerobic exercise, such as walking, swimming, or cycling.
• Ensure you get the sleep you need at night in order to stay awake during the day – it's usually eight hours for men.

Bad habits

• The single most important thing you can do to improve your health is to stop smoking.
• Too much saturated fat in your diet leads to cardiovascular disease – the number one killer of men.
• Heavy drinkers compromise all aspects of their well being.

Information overload

These days it's difficult to get from one end of the week to the other without hearing another health scare reported by the national media. It might be something you read in a newspaper or hear at work, but it all adds up to a lot of often confusing information without any definitive guides. Keep yourself well-informed by investing in authoritative health books and magazines – and utilise the internet. There are several web sites that offer general health advice and are useful as starting points. Two that you might try to begin with are www.medicdirect.co.uk and www.netdoctor.co.uk.

Health check questionnaire

1 **Do you smoke?** It's not good for your lungs and heart, so give it up. Over 120,000 people a year in the UK die from smoking-related diseases. By giving up you could increase your life expectancy by seven to eight years.

2 **Are you exercising?** The least time you should spend exercising is 30 minutes three times a week. Couch potatoes can't afford to ignore the benefits of keeping fit.

3 **Are you always out in the sun?** Ultraviolet radiation from the sun can cause skin cancer, premature ageing, and cataracts. If you're fair-skinned keep out of the sun when it's at its fiercest: between 10am and 4pm. For others make sure you wear a hat, sunglasses, and sun cream with UVB protection, UVA protection, and sunscreen (factor 15 or above).

4 **Do you get enough sleep?** Most of us require eight to nine hours a night.

5 **Are you eating healthily?** If you're not eating a balanced diet you'll store up a lot of problems for later on. Western diets generally contain too much fat and not enough foods rich in starch, fibre, and vitamins (see p.12–21).

6 **How well do you know your body?** See your doctor if there are any worrying symptoms. Study your family's medical history and inform your doctor of any familial conditions.

7 **Do you drink?** If you're drinking over 21 units a week – $5\frac{1}{4}$ litres ($10\frac{1}{2}$ pints), start cutting back (see p.26–27).

8 **Is your blood pressure under control?** High blood pressure is one of the main causes of a stroke and also heart disease. There are no obvious symptoms of high blood pressure.

9 **Do you get stressed?** Try to relax and schedule more time for yourself and your family. Learn to say no at work.

10 **Have you got a doctor?** If not, register with a GP who will give you an initial once-over.

You and your doctor

The chances of dying from a major disease
can be greatly reduced with preventative care,
which means finding a GP you can trust.

Finding a GP

• If you are not registered with a doctor, it's essential that you
contact one as soon as possible. A routine check-up by your
GP not only reveals serious problems, but also gives you
peace of mind.

• When choosing a doctor it's important to have someone that
you're comfortable with. Doctors should be good listeners and
give you their full attention – you certainly shouldn't feel as
though you are being hurried through their surgery. A good
doctor will also explain your illness in terms that you
understand and give reasons, and perhaps alternatives, for an
effective treatment.

• You should see your doctor when minor symptoms persist or
when you experience intense pain or discomfort. You should
always make a point of informing your doctor of any diseases
that run in your family.

• If your doctor thinks it necessary he or she may refer you to
consultants who specialise in one area of medicine, such as
cardiologists for the heart and oncologists for cancer.

Female GPs

While women don't think twice about seeing male doctors
about the most intimate of conditions, a lot of men would
rather remain sick than see a female doctor. It's a pity
because evidence suggests that female doctors are more
patient-centred than their male counterparts. They are
thought to be more communicative, spend more time with
the patient, and are more likely to address concerns that
aren't strictly medical, such as environmental issues.
Evidence also suggests that male patients are twice as
likely to communicate freely with female doctors.

When to seek medical help

1 **Severe headache** Headache with fever, vomiting, stiffness in the neck, aversion to bright lights, and a rash could signify meningitis – a major medical emergency.

2 **Accidents** The obvious injuries, such as broken bones, deep cuts and wounds, bad burns, and major blows to the head should be treated at casualty.

3 **Sudden speech or co-ordination problems** Difficulty in understanding, impaired vision or co-ordination, dizziness or loss of balance, weakness or numbness – down one side of the body especially – are all classic symptoms of a stroke.

4 **Sudden change in heart rate** This may be a warning signal if you're over 50 and there's no obvious reason for it. Also, see your doctor if your pulse races over 120, or falls below 40 and you feel dizzy for no particular reason.

5 **Rectal bleeding** While bright red blood on toilet paper may suggest haemorrhoids (piles), stools that are black and tar-like could indicate more serious upper intestinal bleeding.

6 **Shortness of breath** If it lasts for over half an hour and it's not asthma it could be angina, heart attack, or heart failure.

7 **Non-muscular back pain** If you have pain or discomfort when you urinate, you may have a kidney infection.

8 **Severe abdominal pain** Constant pain for over an hour, especially in the lower right abdomen and accompanied by fever, may mean appendicitis.

9 **Testicular pain** This could indicate a hernia or inflammation of the sperm ducts. Testicular torsion, which is indicated by sudden pain in younger men, requires urgent attention.

10 **Severe chest pain** With sweating and looking grey in colour, this could signify a heart attack, especially if the pain radiates from the central chest to the neck or left arm, and is accompanied by dizziness, nausea, or weakness.

Fighting fatigue

Nearly all of us experience occasional fatigue, and 20 percent of us have consulted a doctor about it. The key to keeping fatigue at bay is to eat the right food and get some exercise.

Symptoms

• You'll feel tired and your head may hurt. You might also have trouble concentrating. Fatigue may lead to depression.
• If you nod off in the mid-afternoon, or you need two alarms to wake you up, you're probably not getting enough sleep.
• Unexplained muscle weakness affecting your movements may be a symptom of something more serious – see your GP.

Causes

• Fatigue can be a symptom of disease, but it's often brought on by lack of sleep, too little exercise, a poor diet, or stress.
• Too little sleep will catch up with you eventually. Most men need at least eight hours sleep every night.
• Long periods of inactivity mean you're not giving your body a chance to oxygenate your blood and revitalise the body.
• A man who hates his job or is bored by it, is a prime candidate for stress; and stress can lead to fatigue and depression.

When to see your doctor

Not all fatigue is caused by lack of sleep, poor nutrition, too much stress, or too little exercise. It can be a symptom of a more serious illness, such as chronic fatigue syndrome, anaemia, thyroid problems, glandular fever, diabetes, lung disease, heart disease, and cancer. Fatigue is also a common symptom of depression. You should see your doctor if your fatigue: doesn't respond to simple measures, such as going to bed earlier; lasts for more than a week; interferes with your life; comes with high fever, dizziness, nausea, vomiting, or bloody stools.

Chronic fatigue syndrome

Chronic fatigue syndrome (CFS) is a debilitating condition that may affect a patient for several years. It's unclear whether the condition is physical or psychological in origin. As well as fatigue, CFS sufferers may experience muscular aches, weakness, poor concentration, memory loss, and communication difficulties. Since these symptoms overlap with many other conditions, a visit to the doctor is recommended. Treatment is usually lots of rest and a gradual build up of exercise levels. Antidepressants are known to help alleviate the symptoms of CFS.

Top five fatigue fighters

1 **Stop smoking** Tobacco contributes to fatigue because it increases your body's need for oxygen, and at the same time decreases your ability to deliver oxygen to the cells.

2 **Watch your weight** If you're overweight you have to make extra physical and mental efforts, which means you're more likely to tire yourself out. Avoid the temptation to go on a crash diet though, as it can slow your metabolism and may make you even more tired.

3 **Examine your diet** Reduce your daily dose of caffeine and minimise your intake of fats and sugars. Go for complex carbohydrates, such as grains and fruit, and drink six to eight glasses of water a day. Take vitamin supplements if there's something lacking in your diet.

4 **Get active** Take the dog for a walk, go rollerskating, learn kung fu – just make sure you get some exercise. It will give you an energy boost and, who knows, you might enjoy it.

5 **Reduce stress** Stress is a symptom of modern life and, if you step back for a moment, you can usually see what's causing it and take steps to control it. You may need to reassess your priorities at work and to check whether you are balancing work and home pressures too finely.

Top tips for extra energy

1 **Energy cycle** Are you a morning person or do you feel most energetic when those around you are taking afternoon naps? Save your most daunting work for when you're feeling most energetic.

2 **Have more sex** Needing to recharge your batteries is not the most romantic reason for sleeping with someone, but an intimate session with a loved one can give you and your partner's energy levels a real boost.

3 **Pursue your passion** If you enjoy something you'll probably be able to find the energy for it. If your job is boring, at least make room in the day to do things you enjoy.

4 **Focus on breakfast** Make sure you have something for breakfast, but lay off the Danish pastries and cappuccinos. Eat cereals with low-fat milk and you'll find that the complex carbohydrates and proteins will keep you going until lunch.

5 **Decline the drink** If you ever drink at lunchtime you'll know the soporific effect alcohol has on you in the afternoon. Alcohol is a depressant that causes drowsiness, so if you're fatigued, give up the booze for a while and see how you feel.

6 **Get some shut-eye** Getting a good night's sleep is a basic but essential requirement for a high-energy lifestyle. Everybody's sleep patterns differ, but you can't teach your body to accept less sleep than it requires. Your sleep also needs to be undisturbed otherwise your body won't feel all its rejuvenating effects.

7 **Get active** If you are in a desk job make sure you include some exercise in your daily routine. Modern life makes it easy to fall into sedentary ways, and if you're not active your body won't be running at optimal levels.

8 **Take time out** Our working days are often organised in big chunks of time, but our bodies function better if we take regular breaks. If you're feeling tired you probably need to spend five minutes away from what you're doing.

Top tips for fighting insomnia

If you toss and turn in the middle of the night, you're among the 33 percent of adults who suffer from insomnia. Try one of the following techniques to help you drift off:

1 **Sleep schedule** Establish a schedule and don't vary it. Ideally you need to go to sleep at the same time every day.

2 **Exercise** Take it in the afternoon, not late in the evening. Leave more time before going to bed after heavy exercise.

3 **Weekend sleeping** Don't sleep in and disrupt your sleep pattern. The quality of the extra sleep is also less than usual.

4 **Relax** Chill for an hour before you go to bed. You can't sleep unless you're calm; an early evening bath is a good idea.

5 **Get up** Watch 24-hour TV or read rather than just watching the clock and waiting for sunrise.

6 **Abstain** Avoid caffeine, nicotine, alcohol, and heavy meals at night. Small snacks can help people relax before bedtime.

Stop the snore

Snoring is caused by the vibration of air passages, especially of the uvula situated at the back of the throat. If you're a persistent snorer try the following:
• Raise the head off the bed by placing blocks under the pillow, and avoid alcohol and pills just before bedtime.
• Use decongestants or a nasal spray to clear chronic congestion, or use the nasal strips that athletes wear.
• Use a humidifier to get rid of dry air.
• Sleep on your side by wedging yourself with a pillow.
• Place a tennis ball in a pocket sewn on the back of your pyjamas to stop you rolling on your back.
• If you're overweight start dieting, and stop smoking.

Headaches

Headaches torment just about all of us at least once a year, and most of the time they are just that, a headache. They may be painful and debilitating but they're rarely a symptom of a serious illness, such as brain tumours, meningitis, or strokes. Headaches that are not caused by an underlying illness are called primary headaches and fall into three categories: cluster, migraine, and tension.

Cluster headache

SYMPTOMS

• Usually strikes over one eye or a temple.
• Cluster pain is sharp and remains steady.
• Nasal congestion may occur and the nose may drip or become blocked on the side that is affected. The eye may also start to water.

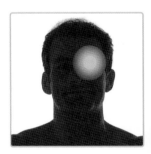

CAUSES

• Little is known about cluster headaches, and they are comparatively rare. One researcher has noted that a majority of sufferers have blue or hazel eyes.
• Many of the men who get cluster headaches tend to be heavy smokers and drinkers. Unfortunately, laying off the tabs and booze doesn't seem to make the headaches go away. However, tabs and booze definitely won't help the symptoms.
• It also doesn't help being male. It is eight times more likely that you will get a cluster headache than a woman. But, again, this is for reasons that as yet remain unclear.

When to see your doctor

If you suffer from persistent cluster or migraine headaches, visit a doctor, who will diagnose you properly and devise a treatment plan. Keep a diary of recurring headaches, including any trigger factors. Occasionally, a headache is a sign of something more serious. Consult your doctor if: your headaches are becoming more severe; they're persisting after treatment; they're accompanied by a fever, vomiting, or a stiff neck; they're accompanied by numbness, tingling, or visual impairment.

Migraine

SYMPTOMS

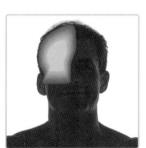

• Migraine headaches usually involve excruciating pain up one side of the head; often emanating from the eye sockets.
• The pain often throbs in time with your heart beat.
• There may be numbness on the side of the face, nausea, and vomiting.
• There may be sensitivity to light, noise, and movement.
• Visual disturbances known as "migraine aura" are often a warning sign.

CAUSES

• Migraines are sometimes known as vascular headaches as they are traditionally believed to be caused by abnormal blood vessel function. Recent research suggests that migraines are caused by abnormalities in the brain's neuronal (nerve) circuits.
• Studies show that 70 to 80 percent of sufferers have a family history of the condition.
• Food may play a role in causing migraines. Some suspect foods that may contribute to migraines include red wine, chocolate, cheese, and caffeine.

Tension headache

SYMPTOMS

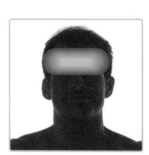

• Characterised by a dull, mild to moderate pain. The pain is steady rather than pounding or throbbing.
• Headaches strike from any direction and there's no exact centre of pain.
• Headaches can cause pain, tension, and pressure in the jaw, upper back, neck, or scalp.

CAUSES

• Tension headaches are more common than cluster headaches or migraines. They account for 70 percent of all headaches and will affect 69 percent of us at some point in our lives.
• Stress or fatigue are most likely to bring on tension headaches. Causes for these headaches are diverse. Eye strain, emotional problems, caffeine withdrawal, grinding your teeth, and even gum chewing can provoke a tension headache.
• Poor posture or sitting in front of your computer for long periods can also contribute to tension headaches.

Who's heading for a headache?

• Many headaches are brought on by bouts of stress. Stress creates muscle tension in the body, and it's this tension that plays a role in many headaches. Pure physical stress caused by bad body posture, for example, can lead directly to a headache.
• Those with a family history of migraine headaches are more likely to suffer themselves.
• Food is thought to play a role in 40 percent of headaches, especially in migraines. Sensitivity varies among people, but there are common culprits.
• You will be more prone to a headache if there are significant fluctuations in your normal eating and sleeping patterns.

Top tips for soothing headaches

If your headaches are prolonged or very painful, make an appointment to see your GP. Otherwise these anti-pain strategies might bring some relief:

1 **Drugs** Painkillers, such as aspirin, ibuprofen, or paracetamol, are usually the first medicines the headache victim reaches for. If they don't work and your headache persists, your next port of call is the doctor. He or she may suggest one of the many prescription drugs available. These may alleviate pain, but bear in mind that men who frequently take painkillers will need ever-larger doses to get the same effects. Some drugs may also cause "rebound" headaches, so if possible you should rely on other ways of managing them.

2 **Exercise** Working yourself into a sweat will release brain chemicals called endorphins, which are powerful painkillers. Always make sure that you are well-hydrated, however, because exercising when you're low on liquids is a common cause of headache.

3 **Relaxation** Distract your mind from your headache by doing a mundane task, or learn specific relaxation and stress-reduction techniques. Try not to be anxious or angry as this will only aggravate your headache.

4 **Old-fashioned ice pack** An ice pack or a reusable frozen gel pack, placed on the source of the headache, can take away the worst of the pain.

5 **Massage** If you have a tension headache, try rubbing your temples for 5–10 minutes then move down to the back of your neck and rub here for a further five minutes or so. Get your partner, or preferably a professional masseur, to give you a stress-releasing massage. It will reduce muscle tightness and alleviate pain.

6 **Peace and quiet** If you're hit unexpectedly by a migraine, try to seek refuge in a quiet, darkened room. Many companies now have sick rooms where you can escape from the hassles and tension of work.

Dizziness and fainting

Often experienced under the influence of
alcohol, dizziness or fainting occur when your
brain receives conflicting messages or not
enough oxygen. Short spells of dizziness are
common and there are plenty of remedies.

Symptoms

• Dizziness describes feelings of light-headedness, lack of
balance, or unsteadiness. It may also involve a feeling
of disorientation and an inability to think clearly.
• Fainting is a brief or partial loss of consciousness.

Causes

• Dizziness is caused by conflicting messages to the brain,
which can arise because of too much alcohol, medications,
stress, anxiety, and illness.
• Occasionally, dizziness can be a sign of a serious ailment.

When to see your doctor

The occasional dizzy spell is usually nothing to worry
about, but if it's accompanied by other symptoms, see a
doctor right away. Warning signs will include numbness,
the inability to speak, double vision, and blindness in one
eye. These symptoms sometimes suggest a stroke. You
should also visit a doctor if:
• Dizziness is accompanied by headaches, loss of hearing,
confusion, or weakness of limbs.
• You also feel hungover.
• You think medication may be causing your dizziness.
• Dizziness lasts more than a few days.
• You've lost consciousness partially or completely.
• Your pulse during a dizzy spell measures less than 40
or more than 120 beats per minute.

What to do if someone faints

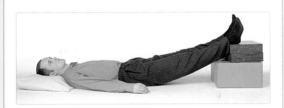

If someone collapses in front of you, don't panic, and don't get them to stand or sit up immediately. Once you've made sure they're breathing normally, lie them down on a flat surface. Then, elevate their feet above the head to get the blood flowing to the heart. Get help if the person doesn't revive within a couple of minutes.

Top tips for combating dizziness

1 **Stay put** If you suddenly feel light-headed or unsteady, keep your head still and lie down and rest. Trying to move around will make it worse.

2 **Move slowly** When you feel ready to stand, first move your eyes, then your arms and legs, and then, slowly, the rest of your body. If you experience swirling sensations (vertigo), sit up and avoid lying down.

3 **T'ai chi** This has been found to help the sense of balance. Also a good night's sleep, a decent diet, and the removal of stress should reduce feelings of dizziness.

4 **Ménière's disease** This condition is recurrent and there is no long-term cure. The symptoms are nausea, spinning sensations, hearing loss, and vomiting. A drug available by prescription will take away its worst effects.

5 **Damaged ears** Dizziness caused by traumatic or degenerative ear damage can be helped by some simple exercises. Try side bends as far as you can go for 20 seconds on each side while sitting on the side of the bed.

Anxiety

Anxiety is an internal alarm system, which alerts us to potential dangers that lurk around the corner. So don't worry too much, a little bit of anxiety is good for you.

Symptoms

Anxiety can make you feel irritable, agitated, or just plain gloomy. Physical symptoms include fatigue, breathlessness, restlessness, insomnia, and muscle tension and soreness. You may also have clammy hands, a racing heart, and hot flushes.

Causes

Harmful anxiety occurs when you start blowing your fears out of proportion. If you start thinking illogically and focus on the negative you will feed your anxiety and eventually you may experience a panic attack when you may hyperventilate, shake, and feel like you're about to faint.

When to see your doctor

Anxiety disorders affect a large proportion of western populations, and they're particularly serious among men because we're less likely than women to seek treatment for anxiety-related conditions. This is unfortunate because therapy, and possibly medication, can treat most cases effectively. You should seek help when your anxiety begins to affect your life. If your work, relationship, family life, or friendships start to suffer, you probably need to seek help. Also seek professional help if your feelings of anxiety continue for over a week, or if you're constantly uncertain about everyday things – such as whether you turned the cooker off or not or if you have your wallet and keys safe. If you are so anxious that you lose weight because of it, you should definitely seek medical help.

Fear of phobias

Does the sight of a snake send a shiver up your spine? Do you break out into a cold sweat at the thought of flying? If so, you have a phobia. Phobias are persistent and irrational fears of particular things or situations. With a simple phobia you may fear one thing, such as snakes or flying. Social phobias may make you feel uneasy in crowds or at parties. The most serious phobias are those that make you fearful of strangers or unfamiliar situations. Therapists treat sufferers of phobias by gradually exposing them to their fear in a controlled situation. This builds up their confidence and eventually the fear recedes. People with a fear of flying, for example, will make initial visits to airports and planes on the ground to raise their comfort levels before taking a small flight on a plane.

Top tips for controlling anxiety

1 **Face your fears** Do this a little at a time, but don't duck out. You'll only confront your fears by staying in the situation that makes you anxious.

2 **Breathing** Breath slowly and deeply, and relax your muscles.

3 **Self analysis** Analyse the way you think. Are you too hard on yourself? Do you play down your good points? Try to re-focus on your positive aspects.

4 **Drinking** Cut down on alcohol and caffeine. Once the euphoria passes your sleep will be disrupted, and you'll feel even more tense. Get physical release through exercise.

5 **Share it** Don't bottle up your emotions. Talk to a family friend or counsellor about your anxieties.

6 **Think positive** Find things that interest you and pursue them. Do good deeds to help you maintain your balance, and keep your eye on life's bigger picture.

Depression

Modern counselling and medicine can help
most people who suffer from depression.
The sad fact is only 10 percent of men would
ever see a GP about it.

Symptoms

Sufferers experience persistent feelings of despair and
hopelessness and they lose interest and pleasure in life. They
may also experience insomnia, constant tiredness, feelings of
guilt or shame, and poor concentration. Physical symptoms
include headaches, stomach pain, and weight gain or loss.

Causes

Some people are particularly prone to depression because of
predisposing factors, such as social circumstances, early life
experiences, and family history. A depressive reaction refers to
negative feelings caused by specific triggers, such as job loss or
divorce. Occasionally a lack of natural light can be the trigger.

When to see your doctor

All of us feel down from time to time, but if you're
suffering from depression your dark days become more
pronounced and last longer. If a very black mood persists
for more than a few days visit your GP who may refer
you to a psychiatrist or psychologist if your depression is
severe. You should get symptoms of depression checked
out because they may be signs of an underlying, serious
disease. If you experience suicidal thoughts, then you
should seek help right away. For most men the subject
remains taboo – they're afraid that others will think them
weak or inadequate if they admit to feelings of
depression. But it's important to seek professional help.
If left unchecked, severe depression can have potentially
fatal consequences.

Treatment

• The severity and duration of depression can be shortened with effective treatment. This varies with each individual but often involves self-help, counselling, and medicine, or all three.
• You can help yourself by exercising, keeping up with friends, sustaining interests, setting realistic goals, and sleeping enough.
• With mild to moderate depression psychological therapy, specifically cognitive and interpersonal therapy, may help.
• There has been a lot of media interest in the antidepressant properties of St John's Wort. This herbal remedy should not be taken with other prescription drugs.
• Antidepressants are often prescribed for moderate to severe depression, while electroconvulsive therapy (ECT) is used in cases of severe depression when other treatments have failed.

Drug therapies

A range of antidepressant drugs are available, but be aware of side effects. There are three common groups:
• Tricyclic antidepressants (TCAs): imipramine, amitriptyline, clomipramine, dothiepin. They help the brain retain pleasure-inducing chemicals. These drugs are prescribed to patients who are likely to benefit from the sedative properties of the medication. Adverse reactions: weight gain, sexual dysfunction, dry mouth, fatigue, confusion, urine retention, constipation, tremors, vision problems, dizziness.
• Selective serotonin re-uptake inhibitors (SSRIs): fluoxetine, paroxetine, sertraline. They help prevent the dissipation of mood-lifting brain chemicals. SSRIs are prescribed to patients who need a non-sedative antidepressant. Adverse reactions: anxiety, headache, dizziness, sleep problems, tremors, gastrointestinal disturbances, frequent urination, decreased sex drive, delayed ejaculation.
• There are new antidepressants available that act as selective serotonin or noradrenaline re-uptake inhibitors: venlasaxine; reboxetine, mirtazapine. These are usually prescribed when other drugs have failed.

Counselling therapies

• Cognitive therapy helps people to recognise and correct depressive thinking. If you make a mistake and think, "That's so typical of me – I'm a hopeless incompetent" it could be the trigger for depression. This is known as thought distortion, which can turn a minor upset into a crisis. Cognitive therapy teaches you to react more positively to negative situations. A better response would be, "OK, I made a mistake, so does everybody and this one's easy to rectify". Cognitive therapy lends itself to self-help as well as counselling sessions.

• Hypnotherapy is now accepted by the medical profession as a useful technique to help people with low esteem. Hypnotic techniques are used to help the patient activate their mental resources in order to achieve realistic goals.

• Psychotherapy has proved to be most beneficial for those with mild to moderate depression. Studies show that the client-therapist relationship is more important than the different types of psychotherapy used. Search for a therapist who you personally like, and who has insight, empathy, patience, and understanding.

• Support groups are useful if you're suffering from depression and you feel very isolated. Support groups can reassure you that you're not alone. They are particularly helpful for drug or alcohol-related depression.

Seasonal affective disorder (SAD)

This is a condition that affects people who experience depressive symptoms during the autumn and winter because of the lack of natural light. It is particularly prevalent in north European countries, for example, where hours of darkness far outweigh those of sunlight. Sunlight is important because it stimulates the body's production of vitamin D and triggers the increase of the mood-lifting chemicals called seratonin and melatonin. If you're prone to SAD it's important that you make the most of what sunlight there is. Even when it's cloudy the sun will have a beneficial effect on your mood, so make sure that you get out of the office during the short winter days.

Top ten ways to boost your mood

1 **Exercise** Strenuous aerobic exercise elevates mood, improves self-esteem, relieves anxiety, improves appetite and sleep, and reawakens interest in sex. Studies show that it helps normalise the chemical imbalances in the brain linked to depression.

2 **Herbal medicines** Some medicinal herbs are reported to have antidepressant effects. St. John's wort (see p.47), kava-kava, and ginkgo may all be beneficial.

3 **Dietary supplements** If you're vitamin-deficient, notably in the Bs, C, folic acid, and biotin, depression may result.

4 **Enjoy yourself** Try not to mope. In mild depression doing fun things can help, so visit a friend, have a massage, get a pet, redecorate, take a class, or go on holiday.

5 **Get away** Organise regular holidays and breaks from work.

6 **Phototherapy** Supplemental artificial light – a half-hour a day in front of a special bright-light appliance – can successfully treat seasonal affective disorder. Escaping to sunnier climes for a mid-winter break creates positive feelings that last for over two weeks afterwards.

7 **Acupuncture** This is now endorsed by the United Nations World Health Organisation as a treatment for depression.

8 **Relaxation, meditation, and visualisation** People who use these therapies often report mood elevation and enhanced feelings of well-being. Visualisation therapy, often used by cancer patients, uses imagery to induce positive thoughts.

9 **Touch** Infants deprived of touch become withdrawn and listless. If touch deprivation continues unchecked the adult is likely to become depressed. Regular massage should help.

10 **Music** Studies have shown that music therapy can help ward off depression. Music therapists may play music while teaching stress-management techniques, or give patients taped music to play on their own.

Fever

You may be sweating, aching, shivering hot and cold, have a headache, and your body may feel like it's coming apart at the seams, but a fever is actually your ally. A high temperature is a sign that your body is working to exterminate harmful invaders. A fever isn't an illness in itself, it's a symptom of an imbalance in the body. A high body temperature enhances the work of your defence mechanisms, especially the action of antibodies and white blood cells.

Symptoms

A fever can be accompanied by specific symptoms, which give you an idea of what's going on in your body. Chills, for example, indicate that something foreign, such as bacteria, has entered the bloodstream. Chills, headache, fatigue, or muscular aches may accompany fever if it's associated with 'flu-like viruses.

Causes

• A wide variety of factors can trigger the symptoms of fever. There are the common viral infections, such as colds and 'flus, and bacterial infections, like salmonella. Stress makes you vulnerable to infections and, therefore, fever.

When to see your doctor

If you experience severe headaches, pain while urinating, diarrhoea, vomiting, or other such significant symptoms with fever, it's time to visit your doctor. If any fever persists for more than a couple of days, then you should call your GP to be on the safe side.

Beyond the norm

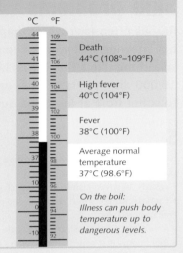

Usually, only very high temperatures will cause serious health problems. But for men with heart problems, a high temperature will put an extra strain on the heart. The metabolic rate rises during a fever, sometimes with an ensuing increase in blood pressure.

Death
44°C (108°–109°F)

High fever
40°C (104°F)

Fever
38°C (100°F)

Average normal temperature
37°C (98.6°F)

*On the boil:
Illness can push body temperature up to dangerous levels.*

How hot are you?

We are told that our normal temperature is 37°C (98.6°F) but this isn't always the case. People's "normal" temperature can vary slightly – it can be as low as 36°C and still be normal. Measure your temperature four times during the day at regular intervals to find your average.

Top tips to beat a fever

1 **Aspirin** The best way to bring down a fever is also the quickest – take an aspirin. Aspirin stops the enzyme that causes your body's internal thermostat to rise. Avoid fluctuations in temperature by taking it at regular intervals.

2 **NSAIDs** Non-steroidal anti-inflammatory drugs, such as ibuprofen, and also paracetamol.

3 **Drink plenty** Fevers will make you sweat, which will lead to dehydration, so make sure you replace lost fluids.

4 **Keep eating** White rice, toast, juice, and fruit will go down well. You could also try taking a lukewarm bath.

Skin problems

Rashes often look worse than they really are, but knowing that won't stop you from scratching like a flea-bitten hound. There are 10,000 different rash types and we're all likely to suffer from at least one during our lives.

Symptoms

How a rash looks and where and when it appears can tell a skin specialist what the problem is:
• A scaly, blistered rash that's very itchy indicates eczema.
• Psoriasis presents itself as thickened patches of inflamed and scaly red skin.
• A belt-like painful rash could indicate shingles.
• Red bumps that appear after exercise mean you've fallen prey to prickly heat (or heat rash).

Causes

• The umbrella term used for most rashes is dermatitis. The most common is contact dermatitis, which happens when skin reacts to a specific substance.
• Some people are prone to eczema, a form of dermatitis often triggered by stress and common in childhood.
• If you are allergic to a type of food it could well be one of the following: chocolate, strawberries, shellfish, nuts, eggs, mushrooms, dairy products, citrus fruits, wheat, tomatoes, and foods containing additives.
• The many causes of dermatitis include illness, allergy, and heat.

When to see your doctor

If your rash is accompanied by other symptoms then visit a doctor. You will also need to pay a call if the rash doesn't clear up after two days or so. Medication can trigger skin complaints, so it's worth checking whether you can switch to another treatment with your GP.

Common problems and cures

• **Eczema** A condition made very irritating by its longevity and intensity. Eczema is triggered by sensitivity to materials, such as soap, dust, or wool, or conditions including stress, dry air, and cold weather. It also tends to be hereditary.

• **Psoriasis** The cause of this distressing condition is unknown but it tends to run in families. During the process of natural skin renewal more skin is produced than is needed, and it accumulates under the old skin forming thick, red scaly patches. There's no definitive cure, but outbreaks can be relieved with appropriate treatment.

• **Shingles** This is caused by a reactivation of the chicken pox virus. A painful belt-like rash appears on one side of the chest, abdomen, legs, or face. Symptoms include fever and fatigue, and there may be blisters and scabs, which can be unbearably uncomfortable. It should clear up in a few weeks, and there are drugs that can relieve the pain.

• **Prickly heat or heat rash** This occurs when sweating clogs the sweat ducts, causing them to break open and leak sweat beneath the skin. The simple remedy is to stay cool.

Top tips to ease that itch

1 **Prevention** Use insect repellents and wear gloves when using potentially rash-causing irritants, such as paint strippers and thinners, and household detergents.

2 **Hydrocortisone** Mild itches can be effectively treated with an over-the-counter emollient. If that doesn't work, you should consult a doctor who may recommend a steroidal cream, such as hydrocortisone.

3 **Baking soda** This will relieve itching, but not the root cause. Mix it into a paste with water, or add it to a cool bath.

4 **Oatmeal** Lotions and soaps often contain oatmeal derivatives. Try putting colloidal oatmeal in your bath.

5 **Tea** Apply tea extract straight to the rash, or via a gauze. Any tea can be used, and you can compound its beneficial effect by applying cream afterwards.

Coughs and sore throats

Humans might be the most successful beings to have ever walked the Earth, but we remain frustratingly susceptible to common hacking coughs and painful sore throats.

Symptoms

A sore throat is caused by an inflammation between your throat and voice box. Coughs can either be dry, hacking coughs or wet ones that help to clear your respiratory tract of mucus.

Causes

• A sore throat can result from a cold or 'flu virus, bacterial infection, glandular fever, and allergens or irritants.
• Coughs are usually caused by colds, 'flu, bronchitis, and irritants, while sneezing is caused by colds and allergies.

When to see your doctor

• Sore throats can usually be traced to a cold, an allergy, 'flu, smoking, or some other irritant. But if a sore throat persists for a week you should visit the doctor as it could indicate glandular fever or something more serious.
• If you think you have an infection caused by bacteria you should see a doctor who may prescribe antibiotics that will reduce the risk of developing other symptoms.
• Persistent sneezing that is not cold or 'flu-related is often hay fever. If it's really annoying, go to a doctor who may prescribe you antihistamines or suggest other over-the-counter remedies to combat the allergy.
• Visit the doctor if any cough lasts longer than a week, or if it is accompanied by symptoms such as wheezing, shortness of breath, or tightness in the chest. Also call your GP if your sputum is thick, brown, or green in colour, and especially if you are coughing up any blood. You may be suffering from pneumonia.

Considering coughs

Coughing isn't always a bad thing. It's a natural function that helps to unblock the airways and keep irritants out of your lungs. A cough is a sudden explosion of air from your lungs, which can bring up phlegm and mucus and eject foreign bodies. You shouldn't suppress a productive cough (one that brings up phlegm) with medications unless it prevents you from sleeping at night. Unproductive coughs are dry hacks that simply irritate your throat. They often occur at the end of a cold, or when you're exposed to irritants, such as high levels of dust or smoke.

Top ways to lose your frog

1 **Expectorants** There are two types of cough medicine. If you have a cough that brings up phlegm and mucus, you should use an expectorant. They contain an ingredient called guaiphenesin that simply thins your mucus, making it easier to cough up the nasties. You will get the same effect by drinking lots of water, fruit juice, or tea. (The positive effects of guaiphenesin have not yet been conclusively demonstrated in clinical trials.)

2 **Suppressants** If you have a hacking dry cough, you will want to suppress it as it's not serving any useful purpose. Medicines containing suppressants – codeine, diphenhydramine, or dextromethorphan – all effectively subdue your body's cough reflex. Of the three, go for dextromethorphan as it doesn't have the side effects of the other two. Codeine is a narcotic that acts directly on your brain; it will suppress coughs all right but it may also cause constipation. Diphenhydramine is an antihistamine and will leave you coughless but also drowsy.

3 **Preparations** Chemists' shelves groan under the weight of hundreds of cough preparations. So how do you know what one is best for you? As long as you choose a medicine with the right active ingredient you'll be fine. Don't just opt for the pricey brand you've seen on TV advertisements. Experts say that the generic medicines are just as good and you'll save yourself some cash at the same time.

Sneezes

• Sneezes really are something to shout about. You might not appreciate them when they catch you unaware in a restaurant, but they are another one of our body's beneficial reflexes.

• A sneeze is an attempt to clear the nose and upper respiratory tract of an irritant. It is triggered when sensitive receptors in the nose are stimulated by inhaled particles or by the swelling of nasal membranes during a cold or hay fever.

• The stimulus travels along nerves to the brainstem, which relays it along the motor nerves to muscles in the chest. The chest muscles convulse and squeeze the lungs. At this point air rushes out of the lungs, throat muscles force most of it towards the nose, and the next thing you know you've sneezed all over your dinner date and fallen off your chair.

• Repeated sneezing is definitely no fun for hay fever sufferers. This is the result of a respiratory allergy to airborne irritants, such as moulds, dust, pollen, and dried animal skin. It can be treated by over-the-counter antihistamines.

Allergies: not to be sneezed at

• Sometimes your body gets carried away in its mission to repel harmful invaders, and it will strike out at harmless things, including pollen, shampoo, or peanuts. These are known as allergens.

• There are three allergy types: contact allergies, which are caused by things you touch, such as wool or cosmetics; food allergies, which happen when something you eat causes a reaction; and airborne or inhalant allergies caused by particles, like pollen or dust.

• Most allergies lead to mild symptoms – sneezing, itching, and coughing, which are annoying but harmless. But for some people, bee stings and food allergies, for example, can lead to anaphylactic shock – a severe allergic reaction that can cause suffocation.

• House dust, pollen, pet dander (dried skin), dust mites, and mould are the most common inhalant allergies. If you can identify the culprit, steer clear of it and try to keep your house as clean as possible.

Sore throats

• It's not surprising that throats get sore. It's the first port of call for all those foreign bodies we suck into our respiratory system. It's usually caused by a virus, bacterium or allergy, but sometimes it's caused by stomach acids that flow backwards into your throat. Your throat may also suffer if it is too dry.

• Sore throats caused by a virus are often accompanied by a runny nose and a cough, and there isn't much you can do about it. These extra symptoms don't always occur with other viral infections, such as glandular fever (the kissing disease).

• A sore throat caused by bacteria is more serious. If it's accompanied by fever, vomiting, white spots on the tonsils, a white or yellow coating on the tongue, and swollen glands in the neck then you may be suffering from a major throat infection. This can be treated with antibiotics as a precaution against rheumatic fever and other complications.

• There is nothing you can do about allergens. If such a particle gets stuck in your throat, your body may decide to attack it there and then.

Top tips to prevent a raw throat

1 **Wash your hands regularly** Most respiratory infections are transmitted by hand-to-hand contact from infected to susceptible people.

2 **Use a humidifier** If you spend much time in a heated room use a humidifier to put moisture back in the air. You can also be kind to your throat by drinking plenty of fluids.

3 **Breathe through your nose** Do this as much as you can and stay away from irritants you're allergic to, such as dust, cat and dog dander, and cigarette smoke.

4 **Gargle** Smooth the symptoms of a viral sore throat by gargling with water containing aspirin or paracetamol, or with warm, salty water.

5 **Sip or suck** Sip hot lemon and honey or take medicated throat lozenges. If nothing has improved after three days, go to your doctor who may take a swab.

Breathing problems

Your lungs and heart are very important
organs, and when things go wrong with them
you know about it. Breathing problems and
chest pains can mean many kinds of problems
from a minor chest infection to a cardiac arrest.

Symptoms

The problem with chest pain is that it's hard to distinguish
one kind from another. It may range from a crushing chest
pain to a sharp constriction in breathing.

Causes

• The deadliest threats to your lungs are cancer and emphysema
(see p.60) for which there are no cures.
• Asthma, thought to be caused by triggers such as dust, occurs
when bronchial tubes go into spasm and restrict air flow.
• Bronchitis is an inflammation of the larger tubes in the
lungs. It's usually caused by bacteria and makes the body
secrete large amounts of mucus, which blocks up airways.
• Symptoms of pneumonia are caused by bacteria or viruses that
eventually cause the lungs' tiny air sacs (alveoli) to fill up with
pus, hindering the transfer of oxygen.
• See page 60 for details of different types of chest pain
connected to other causes.

When to see your doctor

If you have any severe pain in the chest you should see
your GP, or get emergency help if the symptoms fit any
conditions listed on page 60. An accurate description of
your pain will aid the diagnosis. Ask yourself if the pain
is sharp or dull, persistent or sporadic. Does it occur
when you move; is it localised; or does it move around?
What were you doing when the pain started? Try to
describe your breathing; for example, are you wheezing?

What happens during an asthma attack

• Lungs have two roles: to extract oxygen from the atmosphere and to rid the body of carbon dioxide.
• The air we breathe enters the lungs through two major passageways called the bronchi. In the lungs the bronchi separate out into around 250,000 bronchioles, which are ever-decreasing in size. These terminate in alveoli – tiny air sacs covered by a web of capillaries (blood vessels) – where carbon dioxide in oxygen-depleted blood is exchanged for more oxygen before travelling to the heart to be pumped around the body.
• In an asthma attack the bronchial tubes go into spasm and contract, restricting the flow of air. At the same time the bronchial linings swell and secrete mucus, further blocking the airways. This combination makes it difficult for sufferers to at first exhale and then eventually inhale.

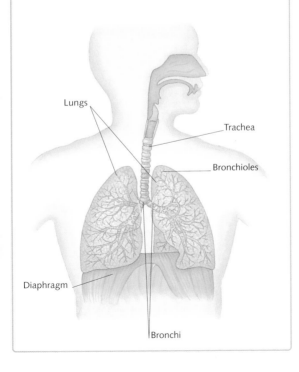

Lungs

Trachea

Bronchioles

Diaphragm

Bronchi

Common breathing and chest problems

• Asthma. Symptoms: chest tightness; quick, shallow breathing; wheezing. Action: see a GP, but seek immediate help if the skin has a blue hue or the person is confused.
• Heart attack. Symptoms: crushing mid-chest pain that may radiate to arms, neck, back, or jaw; sweating; shallow breath; dizziness; nausea. Action: seek emergency help.
• Angina. Symptoms: dull mid-chest pain or pressure under stress. Action: see a GP. Get emergency help if symptoms last more than 10 minutes.
• Anaphylactic shock (see p.56). Symptoms: tightening of chest and throat; wheezing; shortness of breath; itching; swelling; cramping; vomiting. Action: seek emergency help.
• Collapsed lung. Symptoms: sudden chest tightness or pain; shortness of breath. Action: seek emergency help.
• Pleurisy. Symptoms: chest pain, especially when breathing in; fever; headache; dry cough. Action: make an appointment with your GP.
• Bronchitis. Symptoms: coughing up mucus; shortness of breath; fever; chest tightness. Action: drink fluids; take regular paracetamol. If symptoms persist, see a GP.
• Lung cancer; pneumonia; tuberculosis. Symptoms: chest pain; wheezing; shortness of breath; coughing up mucky or bloody sputum; fatigue; weight loss; lack of appetite; night sweats. Action: see a GP immediately.
• Chronic bronchitis; emphysema. Symptoms: persistent coughing; wheezing; shortness of breath. Action: get emergency help if skin turns blue, otherwise see a GP.
• Heartburn. Symptoms: pressure or burning in chest or upper abdomen, especially on a full stomach. Action: take an antacid; remain upright; see a GP if persistent.
• Anxiety; panic attack; hyperventilation. Symptoms: chest tightness and pain; fear; shortness of breath; rapid heartbeat; tingling in hands, feet, or mouth; sweating. Action: deep breathing, and relaxation exercises. See a GP if symptoms recur.
• Pulled muscle; broken rib. Symptoms: pain that worsens when you move, cough, or sneeze. Action: rest and apply an ice pack. See a GP if pain persists.

How to breathe more easily

1 **Quit smoking** Also avoid smoky environments.

2 **Keep it clean** Make your home as dust-free as possible, so keep carpets and soft furnishings to a minimum and banish hairy pets, or at least give them a good, regular trim.

3 **Eat a healthy diet** Make sure your diet contains the recommended daily intake of iron and vitamins A, C, and E.

4 **Moderate exercise** Do some gentle exercise, such as swimming or cycling. If you have asthma and exercise exacerbates it, tell your doctor.

5 **Breathe through your nose** It helps to warm, filter, and humidify the air.

6 **Breathe deeply** Most blood vessels are in the bottom third of the lung, so take deep breaths to transfer more oxygen into your blood. If you take shallow breaths your heart has to beat harder and you have to breathe more frequently to get enough oxygen to your extremities.

What is hyperventilation?

• In times of emotional or physical stress it's quite normal to breathe more quickly. But if your breathing becomes too fast your body will receive an excess of oxygen and a deficit of carbon dioxide. When there are low levels of carbon dioxide in the blood small vessels tend to dilate, and the result is a fall in blood pressure.

• The most common symptoms of hyperventilation are: numbness and tingling in the hands, feet, or mouth area; a pounding heart; chest pain; and shortness of breath. In extreme cases fainting may occur.

• If you are hyperventilating, breathe into a paper bag held closely to your mouth as this will help get carbon dioxide back into your blood. To prevent hyperventilation from happening in the first place, take long, slow breaths – about one every five seconds. Do this as soon as you sense that you are breathing too quickly.

Abdominal problems

The abdomen plays host to so many vital organs that a pain in the "guts" can never be dismissed lightly. So how can you tell whether you've got trapped wind or something serious?

Symptoms

Abdominal pain can be stabbing, dull, continuous, or sporadic, and irregular bowel habits can indicate a problem.

Causes

• Gas can result in sharp pains in the lower abdomen. Other non-serious conditions include heartburn, gastric 'flu, diarrhoea, and constipation.
• Gastritis, an inflammation of the stomach lining, will cause pain in the upper abdomen, while most hernias are accompanied by pain in the lower abdomen.
• Ulcers and appendicitis are both causes of abdominal pain.
• Kidney stones make urinating excruciatingly painful and also cause discomfort on one side of your body, moving towards the groin or abdomen, and blood in urine.
• Emergency conditions that may cause abdominal pain include cardiac arrest, anaphylactic shock, and diabetic emergency.

When to see your doctor

If you have diarrhoea accompanied by fever, chills, vomiting, fainting, or abdominal pain that's not relieved by passing gas and stools, you need to see your GP. If you have blood in your stools, you should see your doctor immediately. If there is any reason to suspect that you have any of the major emergencies listed above, then seek medical help without delay. Other emergencies requiring urgent attention include intestinal obstruction, pancreatitis – inflammation of the pancreas – and an initial attack of gallstones.

What's going on down there?

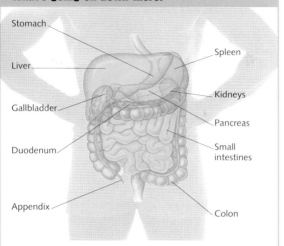

Stomach
Liver
Gallbladder
Duodenum
Appendix
Spleen
Kidneys
Pancreas
Small intestines
Colon

The abdomen is home to the the digestive organs that break down food into a form that your body can use and rid the body of waste matter (see p21):

Stomach Breaks down partially-digested food with acidic gastric juices.

Liver A powerhouse and the busiest part of the body's "food processor" – it detoxifies blood, makes bile (a digestive chemical that breaks down fat), metabolises alcohol, aids in blood clotting, and stores certain vitamins, minerals, and sugar.

Gallbladder Stores bile after it's made by the liver.

Pancreas A large gland that makes digestive enzymes and hormones, such as insulin.

Spleen Filters blood and produces antibodies.

Kidneys Filter waste from the blood.

Appendix Mystery organ – its function is uncertain.

Duodenum Part of the small intestine just after the stomach where bile and enzymes further break down food.

Small intestines Absorb water and nutrients from digested food.

Colon The colon, or large intestine, absorbs water and mineral salts leaving behind waste that forms into stools.

Major abdominal problems

• **Heartburn** Indigestion (or heartburn) occurs when stomach acid flows up into the oesophagus and scorches its tender tissue. Usually, a ring of muscle called the lower oesophageal sphincter stops the digestive juices travelling upwards, but sometimes it doesn't function properly. Smoking, alcohol, and being overweight can all weaken the sphincter muscle, but the main cause of heartburn is over-eating as the stomach has to secrete more acid to break down food. There's a good chance of heartburn if you lie down suddenly after you've eaten.

• **Wind** This unpleasant side-effect is produced when certain difficult-to-digest foods – such as baked beans – are broken down in your intestine. It can cause pain in the lower abdomen and the emissions can be socially embarrassing (or a great source of amusement depending on which social circles you move in).

• **Hernias** These are a protrusion of an organ or tissue through a weak spot in the abdominal muscle. There's a wide range of hernias, none of them pleasant: hiatus hernia (in the upper abdomen), inguinal (in the groin), umbilical (around the navel), and incisional (along surgical incisions). The inguinal version is the most common. Hernia incidence increases with age and they may be triggered by strenuous exercise.

• **Kidney stones** These are caused when minerals build up in kidneys and grow to become stones, which can be as big as peas. The stones move from the kidneys to the bladder and painfully scrape and gouge as they travel through the urethra. Urine may break up the stone or shoot it out of your penis if you're lucky.

• **Ulcers and gastritis** An ulcer is a sore formed when stomach acid burns through the lining of the duodenum (in the majority of cases) while the rest – gastric ulcers – form in the lining of the stomach.

• **Appendicitis** This can occur when hardened faeces clog up the appendix or when the appendix becomes inflamed. If untreated the organ can eventually burst, which can lead to peritonitis.

Top treatments

• **Heartburn** To avoid heartburn, eat less and avoid those foods that can temporarily weaken the sphincter muscle at the bottom of the oesophagus – chocolate, mints, alcohol, and fatty foods are all major culprits. Reducing your weight and giving up smoking will also help keep heartburn at bay. A simple tip is to avoid lying down after you've eaten. Heartburn usually disappears after a short while but if you can't bear the pain, over-the-counter antacids will give temporary relief. There are also medicines that suppress gastric acid or smooth the stomach lining for which it is best to seek your doctor's advice.

• **Wind** If you do suffer a lot from gas – with or without cramping – it may be because you are allergic to lactose, the sugar found in cow and human milk. You can get around lactose intolerance by taking lactose pills, switching to soya milk, or by drinking special, lactose-free milk.

• **Hernias** Hernias mainly affect men and, unfortunately, you can't do much to prevent them. Doctors can usually pop the protruding tissue back into place, but because of the risk of strangulation (when blood flow to the tissue is reduced), they should be surgically repaired as soon as possible. Prior to surgery they can be managed by wearing a truss.

• **Kidney stones** Doctors will usually treat kidney stones with medication and fluids. If a stone can't be passed, the process of litholapaxy will be used to break it up. Due to medical advances only rarely will the surgeon intervene to remove stones. Sometimes a metabolic disorder may be the cause, such as gout. If the disorder is cured, the stones may dissolve naturally.

• **Ulcers and gastritis** The bacterium *Helicobacter pylori* can cause ulcers. If this is diagnosed the infection should be eradicated with antibiotics and acid-suppressing treatment. Stomach irritants should also be avoided.

• **Appendicitis** You can't prevent it but you must get it treated before it bursts – usually 12 to 48 hours after the onset of the symptoms.

Nausea and vomiting

Undoubtedly one of the most unpleasant
symptoms of being ill is throwing up. Often
you have to go with the flow, but there are
ways of stifling and coping with the
technicolour yawn.

Symptoms

Nausea is that queasy feeling that emanates from the pit of
the stomach. If you are nauseous you may salivate excessively,
sweat, and feel weak. Vomiting will result from intense nausea.

Causes

• Prime reasons for nausea and vomiting are eating too much
and drinking more alcohol than your system can handle. Foul
odours, emotional stress and trauma, and certain medications
can also set you off, as can a whole variety of illnesses and
conditions ranging from ulcers, gallstones, and head injuries
to migraine headaches and stomach bugs.
• Motion sickness and food poisoning are also major causes of
nausea and vomiting (see p.68–69).

When to see your doctor

Visit your doctor if you have serious nausea since there
are drugs that can alleviate the problem. If your nausea
persists get an appointment to check for ulcers.
Vomiting alone doesn't usually signify a problem, but
seek medical help quickly if the vomiting is severe,
violent, or lasts more than 24 hours. Seek help quickly
also if there is blood in the vomit or it follows a head
injury. If nausea or vomiting is accompanied by any of
the following symptoms you must alert your GP: chest
pain, palpitations, shortness of breath, severe headache,
exposure to environmental toxins, visual disturbances,
abdominal pain, mid-back pain, or lower chest pain.

Top tips for coping with nausea

1 **Think positive** Sometimes there may be nothing else you can do but "spill your guts". Even as the foul-tasting contents of your stomach come rushing through your throat try to remember that your body is trying to cleanse you.

2 **Try nibbling** If you're feeling nauseated and can't seem to vomit – or you don't want to – try nibbling on crackers, dry toast, or some other bland and starchy food.

3 **Try sipping** Sip on a carbonated drink that's gone flat. Some people swear by Coca-Cola, and it's become so popular as a remedy that you can get an over-the-counter product called Emetrol that's made up of roughly the same ingredients.

4 **Over-the-counter** Another medicine available without prescription is Pepto-Bismol. It is particularly good at calming your stomach if you've had too much alcohol, but it will turn your stools a dark shade of brown.

5 **Delay eating** You may not feel like eating for several hours after being sick. Give your stomach a break and stick to liquids, like water and rehydrating drinks. Liquids will help you stop dehydrating – a common problem with vomiting.

6 **Try sports drinks** Lucozade and other sports drinks are particularly helpful since they contain sodium and potassium and can treat the problem of dehydration more quickly and efficiently than water or other drinks.

7 **Go steady** You will probably feel weak once you have vomited. It's a good idea not to do anything too strenuous for a while. Take it easy and go to bed or lie on the sofa until you can feel some of your strength returning.

8 **Eat mild foods** Once you start feeling better after a bout of vomiting, slowly increase the amount of clear liquids you drink. Eventually you will be able to move onto easy-to-digest foods, such as crackers – once again – or toast, rice, and cooked cereal. If you're still weak you may want to stay on this diet for 12 to 48 hours until the symptoms stop.

Contaminated food

• If you eat food containing harmful microbes your body will eject the contaminated food as vomit or diarrhoea. Germs may multiply on the food both before and after you've eaten it, and the germ type will determine the time between ingestion and the onset of diarrhoea, vomiting, and abdominal cramping.

• If you're healthy, the symptoms should disappear after about six hours, but if your health is already compromised – by stress or diabetes, for example – you should visit a GP.

• Germs to be aware of include: *Salmonella typhimurium*, which is usually caused by uncooked eggs and animal products, notably chicken meat (it will survive being frozen, but thorough cooking will kill it off); *Vibrio parahaemolyticus* is linked to raw seafood and can cause hepatitis in people with existing liver problems; *Escherichia coli* (E-coli) may surface if meat is under-cooked. It may cause death in the very young or old. *Helicobacter pylori* is found in the stomach lining of many middle-aged people. It causes progressive gastritis and is a major cause of ulcers. The organism can be treated with drugs.

How to keep food safe

• Stay away from perishable foods that have been stored for more than two hours between 4–60°C (40–140°F).

•Maintain your freezer below 0°C (-18°F).

• Refrigerate or freeze perishable foods quickly.

• Keep hands and work services clean when preparing food.

• Don't mix meat and vegetables when preparing food, and use different cutting boards.

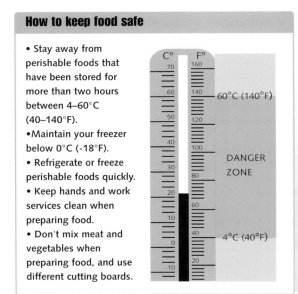

What is motion sickness?

• No one is exactly sure why we suffer from this form of nausea, but we know that it can diminish with age and that some people are more susceptible to it than others.

• Motion (travel) sickness occurs when the body fails to adjust to movement. The inner ear contains fluid-filled canals and sacs called the vestibular system, which keep track of your motion.

• Problems occur when your brain receives conflicting messages from your eyes and your vestibular system. Your eyes may be fixed on a book but if you're reading it on a boat in a gale, the fluid inside your inner ear is sloshing back and forth. The eyes signal to the brain that your body isn't moving, while the inner ear says it is. The confusion may result in dizziness and nausea.

Top tips for coping with motion

1 **Fix your stare** Stare at a fixed point on the horizon rather than at a close object. Avoid looking out of car windows at objects, such as trees and telegraph poles, as you pass.

2 **Choose your seat** Pick a seat where the effect of motion is minimised. In a car or bus this is at or near the front of the vehicle. On a plane, train, or boat the centre is best.

3 **Distract your mind** If you keep it out of your mind, you can forestall some of the dizziness. Anxiety can make it worse.

4 **Hold your head still** Keep it as still as you can, and look around with your eyes, not your head.

5 **Fresh air** Get plenty of it and stay away from foul odours.

6 **Eat first** A modest, low-fat meal before your journey can help. However, a lot of food can produce a lot of vomit.

7 **Avoid drink** Don't mix drink and travel. Steer clear of alcohol and cigarettes as they can compound dizziness.

8 **Medication** Over-the-counter drugs can combat motion sickness. There are also prescription drugs available.

Bowel problems

They may be politely referred to as an "upset stomach" but there's no disguising the discomfort caused by diarrhoea or constipation. The good news is that you can get to the bottom of the problem by eating more fibre.

Symptoms

Frequent toilet trips and loose stools are symptoms of diarrhoea. It can be accompanied by nausea, abdominal pain, or cramps. With constipation, stools are hard, dry, and difficult to pass. Cramping, rectal pain, and anal tearing may occur.

The role of the colon

The colon (large intestine) receives what's left of your food when the small intestine has extracted nutrients from it. The residue is pushed through the colon by muscles contracting about twice an hour. During the trip, which can take from 10 hours to several days, water and mineral salts are absorbed back into the body while harmless bacteria devour digestive enzymes. The end waste should resemble the consistency of heavy cottage cheese.

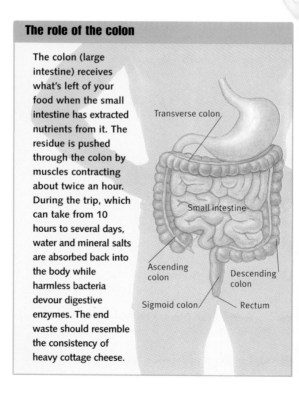

Transverse colon

Small intestine

Ascending colon

Descending colon

Sigmoid colon

Rectum

Causes

• Diarrhoea occurs when the intestinal muscles go into spasm and move your food along too quickly, so that the body cannot absorb water and nutrients.

• Germs often cause spasms – anything from a 'flu virus to microbes in contaminated food – and the diarrhoea is the body's way of ejecting the unwanted guests quickly.

• The spasms may also be triggered by stress, anxiety, spicy food, food allergies or intolerances, and to milk or milk-based products. Eating directly after exercise can also bring on an attack.

• Constipated stools may become hard and dry, and in serious cases they can get stuck in the rectum for long periods. Lack of fibre, taking inadequate exercise, and drinking too little water are some of the usual causes, but travel, stress, antidepressants, painkillers, and antacids that contain aluminium can be to blame as well.

• Not heeding nature's call can also lead to constipation. The longer the stool is in the rectum, the more likely it is to dry making it hard and difficult to pass. So try and keep it regular.

Diverticulitis

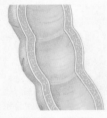 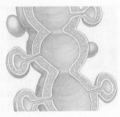

NORMAL COLON   DIVERTICULAE POUCHES

Diverticulae are small, sac-like pouches that form in the wall of the colon. Normally they don't cause any problems, but in around 5 percent of cases they become infected and inflamed, causing a painful and potentially dangerous condition called diverticulitis. It can result in diarrhoea, pain, and fever. A low-fibre diet improves the condition and helps prevent further attacks.

The trots stop here

• Eating healthily, drinking plenty of water, and engaging in regular exercise are all essential if your colon is to produce healthy stools in the long term.

• A healthy diet means eating lots of fruit, vegetables, and grains. These foods ensure that the large intestine is provided with bulk in the form of fibre (see p.19). This indigestible part of plant food speeds the movement of food through the colon.

• The colon, meanwhile, absorbs water and keeps your stools soft and pliable. Nutritionists recommend a daily intake of 20–30g ($^3/_4$–1oz) of fibre, which you can derive from at least five servings of fruit and vegetables and six servings of bread, cereals, and whole grains.

• It's also important to limit the amount of fat you eat, but be wary of low-fat foods as they might come loaded with difficult-to-process sugar.

• Water and other liquids help fibre flush food through the colon and soften stools. Drink lots of fluids, but not too much coffee as caffeine can irritate your colon's lining.

When to see your doctor

Diarrhoea, constipation, cramping, abdominal pain, and other symptoms of colon disorders aren't usually serious and are often caused by unhealthy eating habits or by viruses and other bugs that have found their way into the digestive tract (which runs from the mouth right through to the anus). There are serious diseases, however, that do require urgent medical attention. Do have a check-up if you notice any change in your bowel habits that has persisted for longer than a week. Fever or abdominal pain could indicate something more serious, and if you experience bleeding that's not caused by constipation or a haemorrhoid, something may be afoot, and you definitely need to consult a GP as soon as possible. If the doctor diagnoses diverticulitis, he or she will usually prescribe antibiotics and suggest a low-fibre diet for a while to let the colon rest. Prevention of diverticulitis seems to be linked to a fibre-rich diet.

Bowel disorders and diseases

1 **Irritable bowel syndrome** The symptoms of this common problem are diarrhoea, constipation, or often both; abdominal pain; gas and bloating; and fatigue. The causes are unknown, but a poor diet and stress are the prime suspects. To improve the condition eat healthily, take exercise, or get to the root of what's making you stressed and take positive measures to reduce it.

2 **Ulcerative colitis** Diarrhoea, abdominal pain, and cramping are the main symptoms of this condition and, in rare cases, blood in stools can signify malignant changes in the gut. The cause is unknown but you can treat it by changing your diet, managing stress, taking medication, or having surgery.

3 **Crohn's disease** Chief symptoms are diarrhoea or constipation, abdominal pain, cramping, blood in stools, weight loss, fever, and skin irritation. The causes are unknown but once again a change in diet, stress management, medication, and surgery can help.

4 **Diverticulitis** *(see p.71).* Pain starts in the lower left part of the abdomen, although it can be elsewhere. Diverticulitis may be accompanied by diarrhoea or constipation, nausea, fever, and chills. It's caused by infection of diverticulae, which are small pouches that develop in the wall of the colon. Diverticulitis is treated with antibiotics and a low-fibre diet that enables the colon to rest.

5 **Colon cancer** Symptoms are: persistent diarrhoea or constipation; black, tarry stools or bleeding from the rectum; long, thin stools; persistent feelings of being unable to empty bowels; unexplained fatigue, weight loss, or lack of appetite. The most common cause are polyps (growths) in the colon that become cancerous. Those at most risk of colon cancer – those with a history of it in the family – should get themselves tested as detecting polyps is relatively easy with a sigmoidoscope. Ulcerative colitis can also lead to cancer. Treatment involves the surgical removal of the cancerous colon, possible colostomy, and radiotherapy and chemotherapy to prevent recurrence.

Muscle soreness

The body-conscious male can often be seen in the gym lifting heavy weights in an attempt to impress the ladies. But if he overdoes it, he's more likely to be pulling muscles than the objects of his desire.

Symptoms

• The common variety of stiffness you experience a day or two after an unaccustomed, strenuous bout of exercise is called delayed-onset muscle soreness.

• The extent of your muscle ache or pain depends on what the muscle is and how seriously you've injured it. It can range from a painful, involuntary spasm in the calf muscle to sore back or shoulder muscles caused by overuse, sprain, or bruises.

Causes

• Exercising muscles require extra oxygen, which they receive when blood vessels open up in the muscles to deliver a greater flow. During intense exercise, the blood circulation may not adequately supply enough oxygen. This leads to cramp-like pain in the muscles that disappears when exercise stops.

• When muscles don't get oxygen through the blood they begin to generate energy anaerobically – in the absence of oxygen. When the side-products of this process, such as lactic acid, build up in the muscle it causes soreness.

• Soreness occurs if you over-stretch, strain, or tear your muscles. Tear pain is immediate, while strain soreness is delayed.

When to see your doctor

There's not too much that your doctor can do if you tear or sprain a muscle – it will repair itself eventually. If the pain is persistent, however, it is worth getting it checked out as it may be something more serious, such as a dislocation or a fracture.

Top tips for beating muscle pain

1 **Keep it regular** Muscles that are used regularly have a greater capacity for exercise and are less likely to cause you aches and pains.

2 **Warm up** Before you launch yourself into strenuous exercise make sure you warm up. Gentle jogging or fast walking are good to get your blood flowing and prepare your muscles for rigorous exercise.

3 **Cool down** Gradually ease your muscles out of exercise mode with a five-minute cooling off period. Low-level activity maintains an increased blood flow in the muscle, which helps to wash out some of the toxic side-products that cause soreness. A gradual slowing down will also allow your muscles to return more efficiently to their normal elasticity without causing stiffness.

4 **Drink like a fish** Liquids are vital because your muscles are composed mostly of water, and muscle dehydration is a major cause of cramps and spasms. Make sure you drink before, during, and after exercise. Avoid alcohol and caffeine at all costs, as they're diuretics that boost fluid loss by making you urinate more often.

5 **Antioxidants** Some experts suggest you can protect your muscles by taking reasonable doses of antioxidants, such as vitamin C, vitamin E, and beta-carotene (a form of vitamin A). Body builders use these active compounds because they believe that they combat free radicals (unstable atoms).

6 **Stretching** By stretching out your muscles you're making them more likely to be pliable and free from injury. But don't over do it – once you start feeling discomfort don't stretch any further. You shouldn't stretch your muscles until you've warmed up, either. Some experts believe you should only stretch after a workout.

7 **Don't push too hard** Slowly build up your training programme. Doing too much too early will inevitably lead to muscle soreness. Introduce changes slowly and progressively.

Easing muscle soreness

• Loosen up sore muscles with some very gentle exercise. Do this once you feel the soreness – don't wait for it to subside.
• Frequent, mild stretching exercises will help to bring your sore muscles back to life.
• Wash away aches and pains with a soak in a warm bath.
• Treat your aching muscles to a massage. All types of massage have a therapeutic effect on the nervous and muscular systems.

How muscles work

Muscles are bundles of long, slender cells known as fibres, which are attached to other muscles, bones, or tendons. The body's muscles (of which 639 are named) work autonomously or as part of larger systems that combine the effects of several muscles. A muscle works by contracting and then relaxing; in the same way as a spring shortens when you press it down and springs back up when you let go. Slow-acting muscles are controlled at least in part by hormones, but fast-acting muscles contract in response to independent nerve impulses. As soon as a muscle gets the message to move, the fibres combine glycogen – fuel stored in the muscle – with oxygen. A chemical reaction occurs, which converts the chemical energy into the mechanical energy that allows movement.

Bending the arm at the elbow

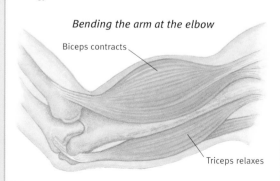

Biceps contracts

Triceps relaxes

Why do we bruise?

• A bruise happens when a knock on the body causes small blood vessels underneath the skin to rupture. The blood flows into the surrounding tissues, there's an increase in the amount of white blood cells, and the area becomes inflamed. The bruise starts out a blueish colour, but as the blood breaks down it turns yellowish-green, and then brown.
• Some men think it's macho to sport a big shiner, but in reality it means they've probably got thin skin. A thinner covering makes it easier to see the escaped blood and fluid. As we get older bruises become more visible because the blood vessels become increasingly fragile.

Three ways to bruise a rib

A bruised rib is the injury made popular by goalkeepers who throw themselves at the feet of onrushing strikers. Bruised ribs can refer to one of three types of injury:
• Your ribs may be literally bruised – unlike other bones, ribs can be bruised through direct contact.
• You may have pulled or torn your intercostal muscles, which are the muscles between the ribs that enable you to breathe in and out.
• Thirdly, you may have a strained or separated joint between a rib and your sternum (breast bone).

Minimising a bruise

To draw attention away from your dubiously-acquired black eye, try one of the following solutions:
• Apply vitamin K cream to make the bruise go away faster. Vitamin K is a blood clot regulator, and research has proved that it can reduce bruising, though nobody seems to know exactly why.
• Apply arnica (a tincture made from dried flower heads). Available from health shops, arnica is well worth trying as it has natural anti-inflammatory properties.
• If arnica doesn't work, employ the tried and tested "frozen bag of peas" approach. A shop-bought cold compress is ideal, although frozen vegetables will work just as well. The aim is to reduce the blood flow to the injury and so minimise swelling.

Joint problems

If you see an old man with a walking stick the chances are that he injured himself playing football in his youth. So be sure to take care of your joints if you want to be walking tall and unassisted in 40 years time.

Symptoms

• There are many different types of joint. Fixed joints are fused during infancy or childhood and hold bones together. Movable joints are more complicated structures made up of ligament, tendon, and cartilage (a strong elastic tissue that covers the ends of bones that would otherwise touch and erode).

• Specialised bone surfaces and fluids also help to lubricate moveable joints and provide cushions against stress. A moveable pivot joint in the neck, for example, allows rotation around a single point, while hinge joints – found in the knees and elbows – allow a swinging backward and forward movement. Ball-and-socket joints of the sort found in the hip are the most flexible, allowing a wide range of movement.

•An unhealthy joint becomes swollen, tender, and stiff. The range of motion is reduced, and any movement possible will be accompanied by pain. Joints suffer a lot of normal wear and tear over time, but specific problems can be caused by sprains, arthritis, tendinitis (inflamed tendons), temporomandibular disorder (problems with the jaw joint), bursitis (inflamed fat pads in joints), and damaged or torn cartilage.

When to see your doctor

If joint pain persists or is severe, see your GP as you may have arthritis or another degenerative disease. Visit the doctor if severe sprains are causing much swelling and pain. Your doctor may need to refer you to an orthopaedic surgeon if your cartilage is damaged. Temporomandibular disorders require prompt attention as does pain that will not respond to drugs, massage, or hot and cold packs.

Sprains and tendinitis

1 Sprains are a common problem caused by the stretching or tearing of a ligament. Joints most likely to suffer a sprain are those that that come under the most stress, such as ankles, knees, and fingers.

• Hold an ice pack on a mild sprain for 15 minutes several times a day for two days. Keep feet elevated while applying ice to lower limbs, and try not to put any weight on the sprain for a day or two. Check out severe sprains with your GP.

2 Tendinitis is the inflammation or damage of a tendon that attaches muscle to bone. Usually the result of trauma or overuse, tendinitis often occurs in the shoulders, ankles, and elbows.

• Apply ice as for sprains, but after a few days an application of moist heat can be beneficial. Anti-inflammatory medications, such as aspirin and ibuprofen, will ease the pain by reducing swelling. Rest the joint area until it feels better, and then only exercise lightly to begin with.

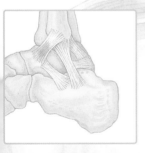

1 Sprains are caused by the stretching or tearing of a ligament that holds bones together. A strain, in contrast, describes an overworked muscle. Joints that undergo the most stress – the ankles, knees, and fingers – are most at risk from sprain.

2 Tendinitis is when a tendon is damaged or torn and becomes inflamed and painful. This often occurs in the shoulder, and is common among tennis players suffering from tendinitis called tennis elbow.

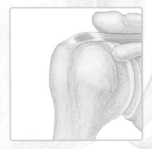

TMD and bursitis

3 The temporomandibular joints connect your lower jawbone to bones on either side of the head, allowing the jaw to move. TMD (temporomandibular disorder) causes the joints to pop, creak, grind, and shoot pain through your head, neck, and shoulders. It occurs when the joints are jarred, such as during a car accident, or when deterioration sets in because of teeth grinding, bad posture, or stress-induced teeth clenching.

• Muscle massage around the jaw joints, hot and cold packs, and anti-inflammatory drugs should all help. If the disorder recurs you should see your GP.

4 Bursitis describes inflammation of the bursae – pads of fat that allow tendons to slide around moving parts of the joints. It occurs most often in joints where constant pressure is applied and is often accompanied by tendinitis.

• Bursitis treatment is the same as for tendinitis – hot and cold packs, gentle massage, and anti-inflammatory drugs.

3 The temporomandibular joints (TMJs) – one on either side of the head – allow the jaw to open, close, and make other movements for eating and speaking. Jarring or deterioration can lead to temporomandibular disorder (TMD).

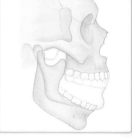

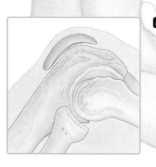

4 Bursae are present, for example, at the tip of the elbow joint, to ease constant friction. When the bursae become inflamed because of unremitting pressure, you get bursitis. This condition on the knee is termed housemaid's knee.

Torn cartilage and arthritis

5 If constant pressure is applied to cartilage the smooth, marble-like tissue will sometimes flake off causing grinding pain. Cartilage can also be damaged by twisting injuries.
• Cartilage won't heal by itself and your GP may suggest orthopaedic treatment.

6 The most common types of arthritis are rheumatoid arthritis, gout, and osteoarthritis. The latter is closely linked to age. Rheumatoid arthritis is potentially the most debilitating and is caused by an immune disorder, which breaks down the cartilage leaving unprotected ends of bones to rub. Gout is a metabolic disorder caused by crystalised uric acid being deposited in joints and can be linked to diet.
• Arthritis is mostly treated with a combination of anti-inflammatory drugs and physiotherapy. The symptoms may be soothed by warm baths, hot and cold packs, and over-the-counter creams containing capsaican.

5 Knee joints are highly complex. A twisted impact, such as a football tackle, is the likely cause of this ruptured cartilage. It won't heal by itself and will require complicated surgery to remove torn cartilage and get the knee functioning again.

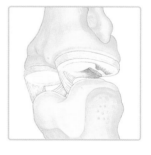

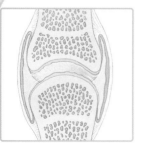

6 Rheumatoid arthritis can be a crippling condition. Inflammation starts in the synovial membrane – the sac that surrounds freely moveable joints and secretes a thick, egg white-like lubricant. It then spreads to the cartilage and bone itself.

Back pain

More working days are lost to back pain than any other ailment. Preventative action and timely treatment, however, will keep you strong and ensure that you never look back.

Symptoms

• Backache is very common and most men will suffer chronic back pain at some point. It can strike anywhere down the length of your spine in one of five regions: cervical (neck) thoracic (middle back); lumbar (lower back); and at the sacral and coccygeal regions at the base of the spine.

• Depending on where it hits and its cause, the pain can range from a steady ache to periodic pain on moving.

Causes

• The main cause of back pain is muscle strain, which is often due to a badly-designed working environment. A bad chair or poor desk height are common problems.

• Other likely causes of back pain are inflamed ligaments, strained tendons, chipped vertebrae, pinched or trapped nerves, cramp, and ruptured vertebral discs. The lumbar region is most vulnerable to pain as it acts as the body's fulcrum.

• Serious forms of back pain include arthritis, osteoporosis, ankylosing spondylitis, spinal stenosis, and spinal tumour.

When to see your doctor

If your back is stopping you from going about your everyday business then get on the 'phone to your GP. Also visit your doctor if a persistent pain gets worse. He or she will be able to prescribe anti-inflammatory or painkilling drugs. You may also be referred to a physiotherapist, an osteopath, or a chiropractor. Make an emergency call if pain is accompanied by a loss of bladder control, weakness, or if you feel numb or tingly.

What gets your back up?

1 **Sprain** If you sprain a back muscle it will feel sore and stiff, and you may experience a sharp pain if you move the wrong way. It often occurs suddenly after an injury or exercise, but it can develop gradually.

2 **Spinal stenosis** The mild pain in the legs that this condition causes worsens when you walk and eases off once you stop or lean forward. Numbness and weak muscles may also occur.

3 **Arthritis** This can occur anywhere along the spine. It's characterised by a steady ache rather than a sharp pain, and stiffness that can extend to the buttocks and thighs.

4 **Osteoporosis** This disease causes the bones to become brittle and more liable to fracture under minor stress. Victims will suffer back pain and posture may become round-shouldered, stooped, or hunched, especially beyond the age of 70. In males it's caused by a decrease in testosterone.

5 **Herniated (slipped) disc** Made of tough fibres and cartilage, vertebral discs are little shock absorbers that fit between the vertebrae to stop the bones grinding against each other. When a disc ruptures, its contents may protrude and pinch spinal nerves. Depending on its position and severity, pain can run from the spine along to the hands and feet. In some lumbar cases there may be a loss of bladder control.

6 **Ankylosing spondylitis** This inflammatory arthritic disease of the spine usually affects men under the age of 40. The joints between the vertebrae become inflamed and tend to fuse together over time. The long list of symptoms includes periodic or frequent lower back or hip pain, pain in the ribs, chest, or neck, and morning stiffness in joints. There may also be eye problems, psoriasis, fatigue, fever, and weight loss.

7 **Spinal tumour** This rare condition is characterised by a persistent pain in the spine which often gets worse at night. Sufferers may experience loss of bladder or bowel control and there is often numbness, tingling, and muscle weakness that gets progressively worse.

Back to life: pain relief

1 **Revised opinions** Not so long ago people with backache were told to take bed rest for seven days. Now experts believe that this is not only bad for business but bad for you, as too much rest can weaken other muscles and interfere with recovery. Also out of vogue is over-reliance on muscle-relaxing drugs, heavy-duty painkillers, and surgery. These methods are still used but usually only in severe cases.

2 **Stop that** If you do strain your back doing something physical, stop. It's amazing how many men shrug off a back strain, carry on lifting, and pay for it twice over later.

3 **Take a break** Have a rest, but not for too long. The National Back Association says that, in most cases, 48 hours rest in bed is better than a week.

4 **Freeze it** Apply an ice pack or bag of frozen peas to the source of pain for 15–20 minutes twice a day. This will decrease painful spasms and help block the pain.

5 **Heat it** After applying ice try using a hot pack, which will also help to reduce the pain.

6 **Pop pills** When severe backache strikes take a pain reliever, such as paracetamol, aspirin, or ibuprofen.

7 **Light exercise** After a moderate rest do some light exercise to loosen up your back, otherwise stiffness will set in.

8 **Go complementary** Try osteopathy or chiropractic for spinal manipulation or Alexander technique for posture training. These therapies are gaining recognition and popularity.

9 **Acupuncture and acupressure** These work by applying pressure (via needles or fingers) to specific points on muscles. This alters the pain messages received by the brain.

10 **Aromatherapy** It's claimed that some essential massage oils help relieve back pain. Massage in general is excellent for relieving muscle tension caused by back problems.

Top tips for preventing back pain

1 **Keep fit** People who exercise regularly are less likely to suffer from back pain. It only takes three or four aerobic sessions a week to keep your back muscles, ligaments, and joints strong and your cardiovascular system in good working order. Low-impact activities, such as walking, cycling, and swimming are best – any strenuous exercise should be preceded by at least a 10 minute warm-up.

2 **Muscle tone** Work on muscles that provide support for your spine, such as your abdomen and buttocks – they take some of the stress off your back when you twist and turn.

3 **Kick the habit** Smoking is bad for your back. For one thing it makes you cough more, which increases the pressure on your intervertebral joints.

4 **Stretch** One way to become more flexible is to join a yoga class. You'll be surprised at how much further you'll be able to stretch in a very short period of time

5 **Sit up straight** Don't be a slouch, especially at work. A good posture means your muscles don't have to work so hard to hold your back up. Aim your buttocks at the point where the chair seat meets the backrest, and keep your feet flat on the floor. Lumbar supports are a good idea if you have a straight-backed chair. Also, make sure your computer screen is just below eye level and that the keyboard allows your hands to be at right angles to your elbows when typing.

6 **Lift carefully** Take special care lifting heavy objects. Lift the object as close to your body as possible, keeping your back straight and your knees bent at all times. Try not to bend forwards at the waist as this will put extra pressure on your lower back. The same rules apply when you're lifting weights in the gym.

7 **Sleep easy** Back pain may be associated with your sleeping position – lying on your stomach, for example, exaggerates the curve of the lower back and twists the neck. Stay on your side or back and make sure you have a firm mattress.

Sports injuries

They might play in the Premiership, but when it comes to injury, professional footballers are easily as vulnerable as you or I. However, there's much we can all do to ease the pain from sports injuries and head off future problems.

Symptoms

• Different sports generate different injuries – obviously you wouldn't suffer the same injury falling off a horse as you would over-stretching for a tennis ball.
• Most running injuries are to the knees, feet, ankles, and legs. Other sports causing lower body injuries are tennis, aerobics, skiing, rugby, and football. Basketball and volleyball are more likely to cause injuries in arms, hands, and fingers.

Causes

• Though impact sports do cause their fair share of injuries, you're more likely to pick up an injury on your own. High velocity movements, such as jumping or pivoting, make your body susceptible to strains and overload injuries.
• The most vulnerable parts of the body are the joints in your back, knees, ankles, hips, shoulders, and elbows. The joints are meeting points for bone, muscle, ligament, cartilage, and tendon – any of which can become damaged.

When to see your doctor

If you think you've broken a bone you should seek medical attention. Broken bones means all fractures, including microscopic breaks known as stress fractures. Stress fractures typically result from high-impact sports, like running and racquet sports. If soft-tissue (tissue other than bone; for example, muscle or tendon) injuries persist for more than 48 hours it could signify a break and you should consult your GP.

DIY sports injury diagnosis

1 **Pulled hamstring** If you don't warm up properly you may experience pain and swelling around the hamstring muscles, which stretch from the buttocks to the knees.

2 **Groin strain** Pain, swelling, and possible bruising on the upper thigh near the nether regions signifies a torn or stretched muscle or tendon.

3 **Achilles tendinitis** The symptoms are tenderness and pain in the heel. It is caused by the inflammation of the Achilles tendon (otherwise known as the Achilles heel), which runs from the calf to the heel. Lack of warming-up or poor shoes can contribute to the condition.

4 **Knee sprain** If you're playing a high-impact sport and experience a pain, swelling, or bruising in the knee region then you've torn or stretched a muscle or tendon.

5 **Ankle sprain** Twisted ankles can involve ligament and muscle tears. The warning signs are pain, swelling, and possibly bruising.

6 **Pulled shoulder** Again, if you have pain, bruising, or swelling, you have probably stretched or torn a muscle or tendon. This is more likely to occur if you're playing racquet sports, softball, golf, or if you're swimming.

7 **Elbow tendinitis** If you experience pain around the elbow that worsens with movement you could be suffering from "tennis or golfer's elbow". This is caused when a tendon becomes inflamed through overuse.

8 **Back strain** If you have a pain, bruising, or swelling in the lower back region you may have stretched or torn a muscle or tendon (see p. 82–85).

9 **Shin splints** If you experience pain in the side or front of the lower leg you may have shin splints. Causes may be tendinitis, inflamed bone covering, or stress fractures.

Top tips for knee injuries

You can give yourself a sporting chance of avoiding injury by paying attention to muscle strength, flexibility, a proper exercise routine, equipment, and mental alertness.

1 **Strength** Even if your chosen pursuit is a non-strength activity, such as golf, cycling, running or tennis, weight training is still recommended because it helps to build up specific muscle groups. Three moderate sessions a week using the right technique, the correct weights, and the right number of repetitions is ideal for most sports, but leave a day in between sessions (*see p.150–151*).

2 **Stretching** Unlike weight training, stretching is something you can do every day, and it helps to maximise the flexibility of your joints and muscles. Start off slowly in any one area and when you have built up a healthy tension hold the stretch for 30 seconds. Don't stretch cold muscles – warm up first – and avoid tugging or bouncing. For stretching exercises see pages 146–147.

3 **The right routine** Get expert instruction if you're not sure which exercises will be appropriate for your chosen sport. Always warm up to reduce the likelihood of muscle tear and help get oxygen into the muscles. Make fluid movements when exercising – jarring motions will increase the rate of wear and tear. Afterwards cool down by doing the same slow, gentle movements you did to warm up. Finish with a quick stretch to prevent your muscles from tightening.

4 **Equipment** The right footwear is crucial. Focus mainly on shock absorption and support. High-top trainers offer ankle support in sports where there is a lot of stopping and starting, such as basketball. Your toes should have about a thumb-width's space at the front, the ball of the foot should fit into the shoe's widest point, and your heel shouldn't slip.

5 **Alertness** Don't switch off during exercise otherwise you'll miss your body's warning signs, including pain. And keep an eye on what you're doing – Steve Cram and Steve Ovett both suffered long-term injuries because they ran into obstacles.

Treatment for sports injuries

Soft-tissue injuries. For injuries affecting tissue other than bone there are four stages of treatment: Rest, apply Ice, Compress, and Elevate (RICE).

• First, avoid any unnecessary movement and remove any tight clothing. If you have an injured limb rest it by placing it on a pillow or soft surface.

• Hold an ice pack to the injured area for about 10 minutes every three hours. If you don't have a shop-bought ice pack or compress to hand, a trusty pack of frozen vegetables does just as well.

• Next compress the area with an elastic bandage, taking care that you don't wrap it so tightly around the injury that you cut off circulation. The bandage should extend above and below the injured area.

• Finally, keep the injured area elevated above the heart using a pillow or clothing.

Fractures If the symptoms of a soft tissue injury don't go away after 48 hours, you may have a fracture so contact your doctor. He or she will ensure that it heals correctly.

Cramp You've seen it at Wembley in numerous cup finals. Ten minutes into extra time and the famous energy-sapping turf claims its first victim of cramp. Clutching his calf in agony a player drops to the floor and waits for a colleague to relieve his pain by wrestling with his leg.

• Muscle cramps, or spasms, occur when the muscle fibres involuntarily contract and freeze in a locked position – as you probably know this can be very, very painful.

• Cramp can strike anywhere but it's most likely to occur in the calf or foot. To stave off cramp drink lots of fluid because dehydration is a known cause. Cramp is also more likely to occur if your muscles are tight when you exercise so make sure you stretch them out properly before taking any kind of physical exercise.

• Cramp often hits you when you're lying in bed. You can reduce the chances of this happening by not tucking in your sheets too tightly and by sleeping on your side.

• To relieve cramp try stretching and massaging the affected area – the pain should soon pass.

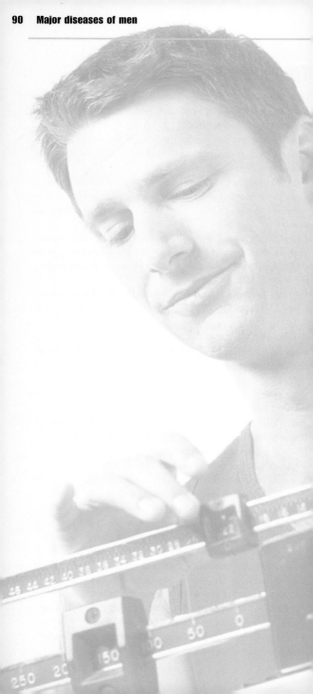

Major diseases of men

Prevention is best
Respiratory diseases
Heart disease
Stroke
Prostate problems
Cancer

Prevention is best

The trouble with the grim reaper is that a lot of men make it too easy for him. Improve your diet and lifestyle and he'll have fewer excuses to come knocking at your door.

Top ten exit routes

- Heart attack. Being male increases your chances here.
- Stroke. Don't smoke if you want to avoid a stroke.
- Cancer of the lung, trachea, and bronchial tubes. Smoking will help ensure that you exit by these routes.
- Emphysema, chronic bronchitis, and other lung problems. Once again, smoking really does kill.
- Pneumonia. This is a catch-all term for a variety of lung-related diseases.
- Traffic accidents. Stop, look, listen, and slow down.
- Suicide. Don't leave it too late to seek help.
- Stomach cancer. A poor diet is a likely cause.
- Colon and rectal cancer: More common as you age.
- Cirrhosis of the liver. Alcohol has the last laugh.

Ducking death

- Most of us have the potential to live to a ripe old age, but only if we choose to. You'll substantially increase your chances of staying healthy in the long-term if you practise the following: eat sensibly; take regular exercise; avoid harmful stresses (physical and psychological); drink alcohol in moderation; and don't smoke.
- Unfortunately, a lot of us will die needlessly because we won't admit to a problem and consult a doctor about it until it's too late. Many men think that going to the doctor is a sign of weakness and they take pride in toughing out an illness themselves. Another reason for avoiding the problem is fear. Many older men especially simply aren't as used to going to the doctor as women are, and the fear of the unknown prevents them from seeking help when they need it.

Side-step the major killers

CIRCULATORY SYSTEM (heart attack and stroke)
- **Risk factors:** smoking; high blood pressure; diabetes; high cholesterol levels; obesity; old age; lifestyle (for example, poor diet, lack of exercise); genetic predisposition; being male
- **Prevention:** stop smoking; eat a low-fat, high-fibre diet, including plenty of fruit and vegetables; lose weight; reduce salt intake; drink alcohol (but only moderately); exercise regularly; reduce stress

RESPIRATORY SYSTEM (chronic bronchitis, lung cancer, emphysema, pneumonia)
- **Risk factors:** smoking; if it runs in the family; urban living; lifestyle; being male
- **Prevention:** stop smoking; avoid pollution, including radon and passive smoking; avoid people with colds or 'flu; exercise regularly; eat fruit and vegetables; avoid stress. See your doctor if you have a chronic cough, if you have trouble breathing, or if you spit up blood

DIGESTIVE TRACT (stomach, colon, and rectal cancers)
- **Risk factors:** old age; lifestyle (for example, a high-fat, low-fibre diet); if it runs in the family; inflammatory bowel disease
- **Prevention:** eat a low-fat, high-fibre diet; avoid salty, smoked, or pickled foods; drink moderately; exercise regularly

PROSTATE GLAND (enlarged, prostate cancer, prostatitis)
- **Risk factors:** age; if it runs in the family; lifestyle (especially diets high in red meat and fat)
- **Prevention:** you can't reduce the size of an enlarged prostate. Decrease your chances of getting prostate cancer by taking exercise and eating a low-fat, high-fibre diet that includes zinc (red tomatoes and soya products are thought to be very beneficial). Cut down on caffeine and alcohol

MENTAL HEALTH (depression, suicide)
- **Risk factors:** stress; alcohol abuse; being young; taking risks; being irrational; ignoring emotional problems
- **Prevention:** recognise and deal with stress; drink moderately; obey common sense; learn to think rationally; acknowledge emotional problems and take action to deal with them

Respiratory diseases

Taking a breath of fresh air isn't as easy as it sounds. Unless you live in remote countryside, every breath you take is likely to suck hundreds of pollutants into your respiratory system.

Who's at risk?

• **Smokers** If you are a smoker you are 22 times more likely to die of lung cancer than a non-smoker, and 10 times more likely to die of bronchitis or emphysema.
• **Passive smokers** If you have to inhale someone's second-hand smoke your chances of dying from lung cancer increase by 30 percent.
• **Urban dwellers** Not only do cities have higher levels of air pollution, they also have higher concentrations of dust, moulds, animal waste, and other allergens. All these irritants increase the likelihood of a respiratory disease, especially asthma. There are also more viruses in the air in urban environments, which means bronchitis and pneumonia are more likely.
• **Older men** Your lungs lose some of their natural elasticity as you get older, making them more vulnerable to disease.
• **Heredity** Genes can be a factor in lung disease.

Breathless facts

• There are 135 million people worldwide suffering from asthma according to the World Health Organisation. This number is expected to increase to 300 million by 2025 in part because of an ageing global population, but also because newly-industrialised countries will be generating more pollutants every year.
• Three million people a year worldwide die from chronic lung diseases, such as emphysema, asthma, and chronic bronchitis.

Common lung problems

Considering the amount of muck we breath in it's not surprising our lungs suffer, although by not smoking we can do all lung problems one major favour.

ASTHMA
• Symptoms: tightness in the chest; breathing difficulties; dry cough; wheezing; occasional asthma attacks
• Causes: colds; allergies to pollen, dust mites, moulds, pets, insects, foods, and so on; hay fever; stress
• Treatment: Avoid source of allergies; drugs (often taken via hand-held inhaling devices); 'flu jabs

BRONCHITIS
• Symptoms: persistent coughing; phlegm
• Causes: smoking; colds and 'flu
• Treatment: quit smoking; avoid pollution; antibiotics; 'flu jabs

EMPHYSEMA
• Symptoms: shortness of breath; coughing
• Causes: smoking, air pollution, genetic predisposition
• Treatment: damage is irreversible, so goal of treatment (drugs, oxygen) is to provide relief and prevent further damage

LUNG CANCER
• Symptoms: coughing; spitting up blood; wheezing; chest pain; weight loss
• Causes: primarily smoking; in rare cases exposure to radon gas or industrial carcinogens, such as asbestos
• Treatment: surgery; radiotherapy; chemotherapy

PLEURISY
• Symptoms: painful breathing; chest pain
• Causes: a symptom of other lung diseases, like pneumonia
• Treatment: treat original cause; drain fluid; painkillers

PNEUMONIA
• Symptoms: shaking; chills; chest pain; coughing (sometimes violent); difficulty breathing; mucus; muscle pain; weakness
• Causes: bacterial or viral infection
• Treatment: antibiotics (for bacterial pneumonia); rest

Top tips for easy breathing

1 **Don't be so shallow** By taking shallow breaths, as most of us do, your lungs are working harder than they need to. Deep breaths are a more efficient way of bringing fresh air into your system and getting rid of stale air.

2 **Avoid pollution** During an average day in the city you're likely to be breathing in a noxious cocktail of carbon dioxide, lead, nitrogen, and ozone. There's little respite indoors with dust mites, viruses, and tobacco smoke.

3 **Minimise your exposure** Avoid pollutants by: not smoking; exercising early in the morning or late in the day when air pollution levels fall; keeping your home and office well ventilated; listening to air pollution reports.

4 **Ventilation is vital** If fresh air isn't circulating, viruses, bacteria, fungi, and moulds will all have the chance to grow. Other sources of air pollution include second-hand cigarette smoke, cleaning solvents, deodorisers, and paint.

5 **Get aerobic** Aerobic exercise helps to increase the efficiency of the network of muscles that make the lungs breathe in and out. It also helps to process oxygen more efficiently.

The perils of smoking

• Cigarettes aren't called cancer sticks for nothing. The tar contains 4000 chemicals, of which 43 cause cancer.
• Levels of carbon monoxide are 10 times higher in smokers than in non-smokers. This toxic gas reduces the amount of oxygen the lungs can carry to the blood.
• The smoker's cough is a symptom of chronic bronchitis, which is caused by irritating chemicals that also affect the immune system, making you more susceptible to disease.
• By smoking you are also inhibiting the lungs' ability to sweep harmful materials out of the lungs, including the carcinogens in tobacco smoke.
• Smoking destroys the elasticity of the alveoli, the tiny air sacs that pass oxygen from the lungs to the blood. Eventually, the alveoli rupture leading to the fatal condition, emphysema.

Top tips for kicking the habit

1 **Quit with a friend** Alternatively, take the plunge and join a support group.

2 **Keep away from smokers** If you're sitting in a pub surrounded by mates offering you cigarettes you're bound to yield to temptation, especially if alcohol's involved.

3 **Go cold turkey** Becoming a social smoker doesn't mean you're any closer to giving up. You'll only annoy your friends when you cadge fags off them. Doctors believe that the best way to break the habit is to stop smoking once and for all.

4 **Take stock** Note when you smoke during the day, and why you smoke. That way you should be able to identify the triggers to avoid. Also, list your reasons for quitting – motivation is a key factor in maintaining your resolve.

5 **Lose smoking paraphernalia** Clean the house, bin the ashtrays, and get your smoky clothes dry-cleaned. Treat your teeth by getting them whitened by the dentist.

6 **Nicotine skin patches** These substitutes allow the quitter to conquer the habitual behavioural aspects of smoking before dealing with the physical symptoms of addiction. Alternatives include chewing gum, oral medication, or counselling.

7 **Coping strategies** You should develop a range of coping strategies if you want to quit. They involve thinking or doing something specific to overcome those moments when you really crave cigarettes. Think about the effort you've invested so far; how much your kids will benefit; your uncle who died from lung cancer. Do leave the pub, go out for a walk, or sit down to play a video game.

7 **Try again** If you do fail on your first attempt, don't worry. You should not feel that you have an addictive personality or are less resolute than others if you don't succeed first time round. Think of an unsuccessful attempt as an exercise in getting to know your habit (for example, understanding when key temptations to smoke arise).

Heart disease

We are more sentimental about our hearts than any other organ, but you would hardly know it from the way most of us treat them. Bad diets, smoking, and lack of exercise are signs of neglect not love.

Understand your heart

The heart is basically a hollow bag of muscle that pumps blood containing oxygen and nutrients around your body. Every day the heart expands and contracts 100,000 times, pumping 33,750 litres (7500 gallons) of blood. When you exercise, your heart beats faster to replenish the cells doing the work with more nutrients and oxygen.

How the heart works

Oxygen-depleted blood enters the right atrium of the heart and is pumped into the right ventricle. From there it is sent to the lungs to be restocked with oxygen. It returns to the left side of the heart before it is finally pumped around the body via a large blood vessel called the aorta.

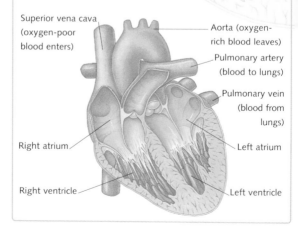

Superior vena cava (oxygen-poor blood enters)

Aorta (oxygen-rich blood leaves)

Pulmonary artery (blood to lungs)

Pulmonary vein (blood from lungs)

Right atrium

Left atrium

Right ventricle

Left ventricle

The circulatory system

Blood is pumped around the body to maintain a supply
of oxygen and nutrients to and remove carbon dioxide
and other wastes from the body's cells. Arteries carry
blood to the cells while veins return blood to the heart.
Capillaries are linked to veins and arteries. These tiny
blood vessels allow the passage of nutrients and waste
between the cells and the arteries and veins.

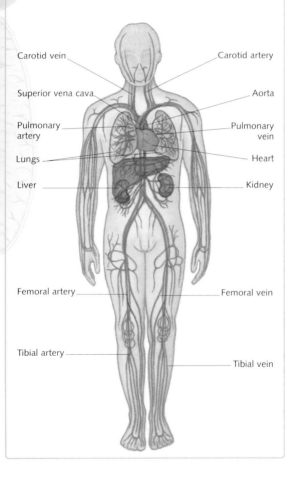

Carotid vein

Superior vena cava

Pulmonary
artery

Lungs

Liver

Femoral artery

Tibial artery

Carotid artery

Aorta

Pulmonary
vein

Heart

Kidney

Femoral vein

Tibial vein

Who's at risk?

There are certain individuals who are more likely to develop
heart disease than others: be it due to lifestyle, age, or genes.

• Smokers
• People with high blood pressure
• Older people: four out of five people who die of heart
attacks are over 65
• Those whose family has a history of heart disease
• Obese people
• People with diabetes
• Stressed executives
• Heavy drinkers

Testing the ticker

• First of all your doctor will examine your heart and chest,
take your blood pressure, and he or she may carry out some
blood tests. The doctor will also look at your personal and family
medical history to see whether heart disease is hereditary.
• Next the doctor may arrange for you to have an
electrocardiogram (ECG) heart trace. It reveals what rate the
heart is beating at and whether you've ever had a heart attack.
• An echocardiogram is an ultrasound scan of your heart. It
can show your doctor how the heart valves are working and
how well blood flows through the heart chambers.
• If you feel chest pains when undertaking strenuous activity
you should take an exercise test. This involves continuously
testing your heart while you run on a treadmill to see how it
copes under pressure.

Is that serious?

• Doctors are often guilty of clouding our understanding of
heart disease by using complicated terminology. Some terms
to remember include:
• Atherosclerosis (hardening of the arteries). This condition
occurs when cholesterol and other substances build up on the
inner walls of arteries. When those arteries supplying blood to
the heart are clogged you've got heart disease.
• Hypertension is otherwise known as high blood pressure.
• Coronary heart disease is another term for heart disease.

Heart and circulatory problems

ANGINA
Symptoms: Chest pain felt during exercise or stress. Pain often
radiates from the breastbone towards the left shoulder and arm
Causes: Heart disease
Treatment: Drugs or surgery

ARRHYTHMIA
Symptoms: Fluttering sensations in the sufferer's chest or neck.
In more severe cases there may be fatigue, light-headedness,
unconsciousness, or even death
Causes: Misfiring of the heart's electrical system, often caused
by high blood pressure, ageing, or atherosclerosis
Treatment: Medications; various non-surgical techniques;
implanting a pacemaker in serious cases

CARDIAC ARREST
Symptoms: Loss of heart function leading rapidly to death
Causes: All heart conditions can cause a cardiac arrest. Unlike
in a heart attack, the heart muscle doesn't die from a lack of
blood supply. It stops because of a disruption in the electrical
signals that govern its beating (arrhythmia)
Treatment: Cardio-pulmonary resuscitation (CPR) within minutes

HEART ATTACK
Symptoms: Feelings of heaviness, burning, or pressure in the
middle of the chest, sometimes spreading to the left arm and
up into the neck or jaw. Often the pain is uncomfortable rather
than severe and victims may be unaware of an attack. Sweating,
nausea, pallor, or shortness of breath are also symptoms
Causes: Blockage of coronary arteries caused by
atherosclerosis. 85 percent of heart attacks are caused when
an artery in the heart, already clogged by cholesterol, becomes
blocked off entirely by a blood clot
Treatment: CPR; emergency medical attention; drugs

HIGH BLOOD PRESSURE
Symptoms: Possible pain at back of head; no others
Causes: Atherosclerosis is a factor; rarely kidney disease
Treatment: Reduction in salt and alcohol intake; more exercise;
weight loss, life-long medication

Staying hale and hearty

• Don't smoke. Men with high cholesterol levels are twice as likely to have a heart attack if they smoke.

• Avoid saturated fats as they clog up arteries faster than any other food. Be prepared to cut back on fried foods, meat, whole dairy products, egg yolks, and offal meats. Stock your kitchen cupboards up with plenty of fruit, vegetables, and whole grains instead.

• Exercise. Since your heart is a muscle it needs a regular work out just like the other muscles in your body. You don't have to run a marathon – a 20-minute walk or a gardening session five times a week should be enough to keep your ticker in order.

Time to de-stress

Experts believe that stress, anger, and anxiety all increase your chances of suffering from heart disease or having a heart attack. Although everybody experiences stress in their lives some people manage it more effectively than others. Try the following suggestions to cope more easily with the stresses and strains in your life: learn relaxation techniques; practise meditation; take up yoga or t'ai chi; find a relaxing hobby; visit a counsellor; take regular holidays; visit your GP about medication (as a last resort).

When to see your doctor

Don't wait until you are at death's door to see a doctor about any severe chest pains. The following symptoms need medical attention:

• Discomfort in the chest area after exercise

• Feelings of pressure on the chest or burning and squeezing sensations (the discomfort may also be felt in the arms or neck)

• If you're having difficulty breathing it could be a sign that the heart is not pumping oxygen around your body hard enough

Blood pressure

Have you ever wondered why there are two readings when you have your blood pressure taken? The top reading, called the systolic pressure, indicates the pressure of the blood when your heart is contracting to push blood around the body. The lower reading, diastolic pressure, represents the pressure of your heart when it relaxes. If the systolic number is high it means your heart is probably working too hard. A high reading of the diastolic number means that arteries aren't getting the break they need. If either pressure reading is high it could be a sign of clogged arteries. A reading of less than 140 over 90 indicates normal adult blood pressure.

Four steps to a clogged artery

The heart pumps blood through coronary arteries surrounding the heart's surface. The clogging of these arteries is the most common form of heart disease. The diagrams below illustrate how such arteries get clogged.

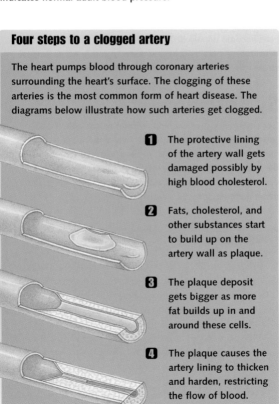

1 The protective lining of the artery wall gets damaged possibly by high blood cholesterol.

2 Fats, cholesterol, and other substances start to build up on the artery wall as plaque.

3 The plaque deposit gets bigger as more fat builds up in and around these cells.

4 The plaque causes the artery lining to thicken and harden, restricting the flow of blood.

Stroke

Strokes are the second most common cause of death in men today, and because the symptoms of a stroke are easy to ignore it's a very effective killer. Many strokes can be prevented by healthy living.

Causes

Strokes happen when there's an interruption in the flow of blood into the brain. They occur when blood clots form or blood vessels rupture. The cells that are no longer receiving blood start to die and the parts of the body controlled by these cells become impaired. The consequences of this can be devastating: paralysis, loss of speech, and in 40 percent of stroke cases, death.

Symptoms

Get emergency medical help as soon as possible if you experience a combination of the following: weakness; numbness in the face, arms, or legs (especially on one side of the body); blurry vision or loss of vision (especially in one eye); dizziness or loss of balance; difficulty speaking and understanding speech; severe headache.

Who's at risk?

- Those who have a family history of strokes.
- Those with thick blood, for example with high red blood cell counts, are more likely to have clots.
- Older people – two-thirds of victims are over 65.
- Men are 30 percent more prone than women.
- People who've already had a stroke or heart attack.
- People with high blood pressure, high cholesterol levels, hardening of the arteries, or diabetes; smokers; the physically inactive; the obese; or heavy drinkers.
- People who've experienced an irregular heartbeat.

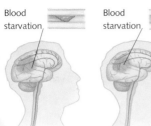
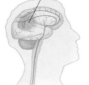
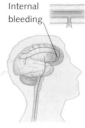

Blood starvation

Blood starvation

Internal bleeding

Clot develops on blood vessel wall

Clot arrives from elsewhere in the body

Blood vessel wall ruptures locally

Three main causes of stroke

1 **Blockages** The most common reason for a stroke is when a clot blocks the flow of blood through an artery or vein in the brain. The clot can either be fixed on the wall of the blood vessel or be carried by the blood from another part of the body. The brain cells that are no longer being supplied by blood die, affecting the part of the body they were controlling.

2 **Rupture** Ruptures cause the haemorrhagic strokes that give boxing a bad name. They occur when an artery or vein in the brain swells or breaks, and they are caused by high blood pressure or a weak spot on a blood vessel wall. Weak spots can be aneurysms (balloon-like swellings in arteries), which can be present at birth. Strokes are also caused by hardening of the arteries (atherosclerosis) or high blood pressure. As well as the danger posed by the loss of blood, burst blood vessels put pressure on the tightly-crammed cavity of the brain, affecting the brain's functions. Many haemorrhagic stroke victims make a full recovery because the injured tissue can recover when the pressure is relieved.

3 **Son of stroke** Mini-strokes, or transient ischaemic attacks (TIAs), can be lifesavers because they alert you to the possibility of a major stroke. This buys you the time to visit your doctor who may offer you advice or prescribe you drugs. TIAs occur when arteries to the brain are briefly blocked. If a blockage lasts for more than 24 hours it's defined as a stroke. The symptoms of mini-stroke leave no permanent damage once the clot breaks up.

Prostate problems

Otherwise known as the "worrisome walnut", the prostate gland has an alarming tendency to develop cancer and, for some reason, it grows bigger as you get older.

The major threats

• **Prostate cancer** (*see p.109*). There are no symptoms during the early stages. Eventually problems with urination will arise including the constant feeling you need to urinate and dribbling after urinating. Advanced cases may lead to impotence, swollen lymph nodes in the groin area, blood in urine, pain in the pelvis, and bone pain. Causes are unknown but genetics and diet may be factors. Depending on the stage of the disease drugs, surgery, or radiotherapy may be used as treatment.
• **Enlarged prostate** The prostate gets bigger as you reach middle age (*see p.108*). Most men get used to the irritation caused by an enlarged prostate but some elect to take drugs or have surgery.
• **Prostate infections** Symptoms are fever, severe pain in lower abdomen and groin, chills, penile discharge, and painful urination. These are caused by bacterial and viral infections; inflammation of the urinary tract; sexually-transmitted diseases; and stress. Bacterial infection is treated with antibiotics, and non-bacterial infections with warm baths and ibuprofen.

Who's at risk?

• Men over 50, who are also more likely to have an enlarged prostate.
• Males who are genetically predisposed (who have a history of the cancer in their family).
• Males living in Europe and North America are more likely to suffer than Asians and South Americans because of poorer diet.
• Red meat eaters.

Finding the walnut

The prostate gland is playing hide and seek between the bladder and the penis. To complicate matters it's also wrapped around the urethra. It needs to sit in this precarious position because it plays an important part in reproduction. Without the prostate gland your sperm probably wouldn't reach its final destination, as the gland manufactures 90 percent of the milky seminal fluid you ejaculate. The mechanics are simple. When you are sexually aroused your sperm travels from your testicles through a tube called the vas deferens. The sperm joins the urethra at the level of your prostate gland, where it mixes with the prostate's semen prior to being fired off.

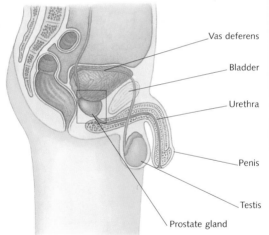

Vas deferens

Bladder

Urethra

Penis

Testis

Prostate gland

The urethra (along which both sperm and urine travel) passes straight through the prostate gland. This is where sperm meets up with semen before it leaves the penis.

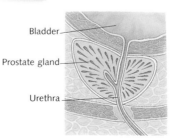

Bladder

Prostate gland

Urethra

Growing pains

• When you consider that the prostate gland can grow to be the size of an orange it's not surprising that it causes problems for the urethra that passes through it.

• The first figure (*see below*) shows a healthy prostate with a wide, healthy "boulevard" of a urethra.

• The second figure shows how a benign growth of tissue narrows the channel. This is known as benign prostatic hyperplasia (BPH). The severity of BPH varies among individuals and so does the treatment. Many doctors recommend a watch and wait strategy, which means regular check-ups to see if the condition deteriorates.

• In the third figure the condition has deteriorated so far that only a small part of the urethra remains unblocked.

What happens when a prostate grows

The first figure shows a healthy prostate gland. The urethra (the tube that carries both sperm and urine through the penis) is wide and unblocked.

Urethra

Healthy prostate tissue

The prostate gland starts to grow in size leading to benign prostatic hyperplasia, or BPH, in which the prostate squeezes the urethra (benign means non-cancerous and hyperplasia means increased cell growth).

Benign growth narrows urethra

The benign prostatic hyperplasia may become so severe that only a very small part of the urethra remains unblocked. This leads to problems with urination.

Urethra is almost closed

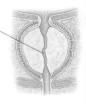

Prostate cancer

• No one is quite sure what causes prostate cancer but poor diet is a prime suspect. Studies suggest that a diet low in fat and cholesterol can help prevent the disease. Foods that scientists have identified as being particularly beneficial include red tomatoes and soya products. If you are deficient in vitamins A, C, and E, you may also be more vulnerable.

• If you have symptoms of the disease or a history of it in the family visit your GP who may give you a blood test or a digital rectal examination. If you catch it early enough the chances of survival are almost 100 percent.

• As most tumours grow slowly, men often forego surgery because it can cause impotence. A surgical technique has recently been developed that preserves potency, but it is more effective for men in their 40s and 50s than for those in their 60s and older.

Top tips for a healthy prostate

1 **Keep the pressure off** Life might begin at 40, but it is also the age when your prostate starts causing you problems. When your prostate gland gets larger you can help to keep the pressure off the urethra in one of three ways: urinate regularly, don't stay seated in one place for too long, and – hurrah – have more sex.

2 **Get physical** Exercise is not only good for your heart it also helps to keep the prostate in trim. Men who exercise regularly are less likely to have prostate problems, so try and fit in three 30-minute sessions a week.

3 **Eat well** Give your prostate a fighting chance by eating a low-fat, low-cholesterol diet. Be sure also to eat foods rich in vitamins A, C, and E. A wide variety of fruit and vegetables, especially green leafy vegetables such as spinach, kale, and broccoli, will ensure a good supply. Zinc may be another ally. You'll find it in oysters, nuts, wheat germ, bran, eggs, pumpkin seeds, chicken, peas, and lentils.

Cancer

Cancer is no longer the out-and-out killer it once was. Advanced techniques in detection and surgery can help to conquer even advanced tumours. You can do your bit by living a lifestyle that discourages cancer cells from taking up residency in the first place.

The dreaded disease

• While an absolute cure for cancer remains tantalisingly out of reach, medical advances are giving us a much better chance of beating cancer than ever before.

• There are over 100 different forms of cancer and they all have one thing in common: renegade cells grow and multiply, overrunning the body's natural control mechanisms. The cancer cells start to spread, attacking healthy tissues, blocking passageways, eroding bone, and destroying nerves.

• There are certain cancers we can do nothing about, but you can reduce the odds of getting most types of cancer by pursuing a healthy lifestyle. One specialist has estimated that changes in lifestyle could reduce the chances of cancer by 70 percent.

• Having a regular private medical check-up can also greatly increase your chances of beating cancer. Malignant growths can be spotted early on and be treated before they spread to other areas.

Who's at risk?

Smokers already know that cigarettes cause 85 percent of lung cancers and are a major cause of mouth, oesophageal, throat, pancreas, and bladder cancer. Those who eat too much fat and not enough fruit and vegetables are susceptible to colon and stomach cancer, while heavy drinkers are prone to liver, mouth, throat, and oesophageal cancer. Cancer is more likely in those exposed to carcinogens and excess sun.

What is a tumour?

A tumour is simply an abnormal growth that serves no purpose. They are either benign (non-cancerous) or malignant (cancerous). When tumours grow they destroy healthy surrounding tissue. Malignant cells will eventually metastasise – migrate out through the blood stream or lymphatic system and form tumours in other parts of the body. To have a reasonable chance of surviving cancer, growths must be detected before they metastasise. Tumours can grow very slowly and they may not metastasise for years, but unfortunately people only generally detect cancer symptoms once this stage has been reached. That's one very good reason why it's best to avoid carcinogens and live healthily.

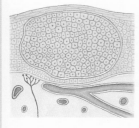

A benign tumour grows but does not migrate to other parts of the body.

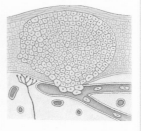

A malignant tumour grows and migrates to other parts of the body.

Watch yourself

Cancer symptoms are wide-ranging and all could indicate something else. Symptoms that you should get checked out include: a change in bowel or bladder habits; sores that don't heal; mole or wart changes; unusual bleeding or discharges; lumps; persistent indigestion; difficulty in swallowing; persistent hoarseness, cough, or low-grade fever; unusual tiredness; constant headaches or pains; excessive bruising; pallor; loss of appetite or weight.

Lung cancer

As in most cancers the appearance of symptoms usually mean that the disease is fairly advanced. Watch out particularly for persistent coughs and blood in the phlegm. Other symptoms include chronic bronchitis, chest pains, and breathlessness. Smoking is the biggest cause of lung cancer by far – you are much more likely to develop it if you smoke. Other causes include exposure to carcinogenic chemical and industrial substances, such as arsenic, radon, and asbestos, which you should endeavour to steer clear of. The number one prevention method is simple – quit smoking (passive or otherwise). You should also moderate your alcohol intake. To build up protection against lung cancer eat foods containing vitamins A, C, and E – the best sources of which are fruit and vegetables. Once diagnosed, lung cancer is managed with surgery, radiotherapy, and chemotherapy.

Liver cancer

Loss of weight and appetite, and pain and swelling in the upper abdomen are all symptoms of liver cancer. Jaundice or anaemia may also be present. There is a blood test that can reveal increased enzyme levels that indicate the presence of liver cancer. Liver cancer by itself is rare; usually the malignancy will have spread from another part of the body. In the developed world liver cancer is usually caused by alcohol-induced cirrhosis, while in Asia and Africa chronic infection with a hepatitis virus is the more likely cause. In some countries moulds and fungi in certain foods can trigger liver cancer. Unless you're an alcoholic you will almost certainly avoid liver cancer if you don't catch hepatitis. Keep clear of hepatitis infection by declining unsafe sex and avoiding dirty hypodermic needles. There is a vaccine for hepatitis B for those at risk, but not one for hepatitis C. Most liver cancer in the West is caused by heavy drinking, so limit yourself to three drinks a day.

Colon cancer

Any sign of blood in the stools must be checked out by your GP – it may well indicate piles, but it could mean cancer. Other colon cancer symptoms include pain in the lower abdomen and unexplained weight loss. If changes in your bowel habits persist for more than a week it could be a sign. Polyps, or wart-like growths, in the colon usually cause colon cancer. The disease is genetic, so find out if there's a family history of it and speak to your doctor about getting regularly tested. If you have inflammatory bowel disease you are slightly more likely to develop colon cancer. Doctors will look for microscopic traces of blood in your stool, and if they suspect polyps they may recommend tests, such as a rectal exam, proctoscopy, or colonoscopy. Your best chance of preventing colon cancer is to eat plenty of fibre, found in whole grains, pulses, fruit, and vegetables. It's managed by surgery, radiotherapy, and chemotherapy.

Stomach cancer

This is one of the more dangerous cancers as symptoms don't show themselves until the disease is well established. They include vague discomfort in the abdomen, a sense of fullness in the upper abdomen, even after small meals, and, in later stages, heartburn, indigestion, or ulcer-like symptoms, vomiting and nausea, or loss of weight. The exact cause of stomach cancer is unclear, but researchers have identified smoked foods, salted meat and fish, pickled vegetables, and starch as risky. Smoking and alcohol also increase the risk of stomach cancer. Men are twice as likely to develop the disease as women. Eating foods containing vitamins A and C lowers the risk, as does eating plenty of bread, cereals, pasta, rice, and beans. Be on your guard against stomach cancer if your family has a history of it or, for reasons as yet unknown, you have blood type A. Surgery, radiotherapy, and chemotherapy are used to keep stomach cancer in check.

Skin cancer

Symptoms to watch out for include any change in the
skin, especially the size, colour, or shape of a mole or
other dark spot or growth. Scaliness, oozing, bleeding,
itchiness, tenderness, or pain could all be signs of the
disease. Exposing the skin to dangerous levels of
ultraviolet radiation in sunlight is a well-known cause of
skin cancer. Men with fair complexions are particularly
vulnerable. You'll also put yourself at risk if you expose
yourself to substances such as coal tar, pitch, creosote,
and arsenic. Skin cancer can be genetic. To dramatically
reduce the risks, protect yourself from the sun. Or as
Australians would say, "slip, slap, slop" – slip on a long-
sleeved shirt, slap on some sunblock, and slop on a hat.
The condition can be treated by surgery; radiotherapy;
cryosurgery (tissue destruction by freezing); electro-
desiccation (tissue destruction by heat); or laser therapy.
Chemotherapy or anti-cancer vaccines are used rarely.

Testicular cancer

The most common symptom is a small, hard lump about
the size of a pea on one of the testicles. Soreness or
heaviness in the scrotum or scrotal swelling are other
signs of testicular cancer. All these symptoms may
indicate only bacterial infection or cysts. This is another
cancer where the "cause unknown" box remains ticked.
It usually affects men aged 15–39 and it may be linked
to the hormonal changes that occur at puberty. Men
who experienced an undescended testicle have a greater
chance of developing the disease, as have those with a
history of the cancer in their family. As testicular cancer
has such a high cure rate – 90 percent – it's foolish not
to check yourself regularly. Every month or so look for
lumps, swelling, hardening, or anything that looks
unusual. It's best to do it after a bath or shower when
the scrotum is relaxed. There's no need to bring tears to
your eyes, just gently roll the testicles between your
thumb and fingers.

Prostate cancer

There are no symptoms at first but you'll eventually
have problems with urination – frequent and poor flow
and the need to pee just after you have. The cause is
uncertain but low-fat, low-cholesterol diets are thought
to aid prevention. If cancer is deemed life-threatening,
chemotherapy, radiotherapy, and surgery may be used.
To help prevent prostate cancer exercise regularly and
eat plenty of fruit and vegetables. Also make sure you
urinate regularly, don't remain seated for too long, and
have as much sex as you can.

Top tips for limiting cancer

1 **Stay clear of carcinogens** At least half of all cancer deaths
are caused because of prolonged exposure to a carcinogen.
Tobacco is the biggest villain. The likelihood of developing
cancer is proportional to how long you are exposed to the
carcinogen and at what intensity.

2 **Improve your diet** Stomach cancer has actually declined in
industrialised countries in the last 30 years. Epidemiologists
put this down to the decline in consumption of cured,
preserved, and salted foods, and an increase in the
consumption of fresh fruit and vegetables.

3 **Check your family history** If you have relatives who have
had cancer you should talk to your GP about how to reduce
your chances of carrying on the family tradition. Your doctor
should ensure you have regular tests.

4 **Cut back on the booze** The link is uncertain, but you
are more likely to develop cancer if you drink heavily.
This is especially so in the case of liver cancer.

5 **Give yourself the once over** You may be able
to spot the tumours of some
cancers yourself, especially in
the case of testicular and
skin cancer.

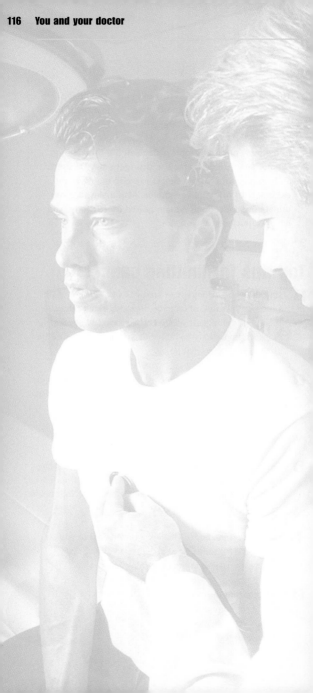

You and your doctor

Getting help
The good GP guide
Complementary therapies
Drug treatments

Getting help

Without regular help from medical professionals you'll be ill-equipped to cope with health problems that are inevitable as you age.

Top reasons to see a GP

- A cough that won't go away
- Chest pain, breathing problems, or high blood pressure
- Problems with urination or erection
- Fever, earache, sore throat, or skin rash
- Visual problems
- Persistent back or joint pains
- Nasal congestion or headache
- Abdominal pain
- Depression or insomnia
- Unexplained weight loss

Symptoms you can't ignore

- Chest pain may indicate heartburn, but it could be a heart problem and only your doctor will know for sure. The symptoms of heart disease range from crushing upper body pain that lasts for several minutes to vague chest discomfort.
- If you're struggling for breath contact your doctor.
- If dizziness is severe or occurs regularly seek prompt medical attention as it could be a sign of a stroke.
- Failure to get an erection is a justifiable – and reasonably common – reason to see a doctor.
- See your doctor if you spot blood in urine or stools or if you're having to get up frequently at night to pee.
- Sudden or unexpected weight loss.
- Excessive thirst and urination may indicate diabetes.
- If a wound is taking longer than usual to heal it could indicate problems with the immune system.
- If an illness is lingering see a doctor even if the symptoms are mild.

Communicating with your doctor

Unlike women, men aren't very good at telling doctors about their ailments. Doctors won't stand much of a chance of making a correct diagnosis if the patient stands silent while being examined. A study found that in a 15-minute session women typically ask six questions, while men fail to ask a single one. Men are particularly reluctant to discuss sexual matters, which could cost them dearly because sexual functioning is a good barometer of general health. And it's no good waiting for the doctor to guess what's wrong. Few of them ask questions – they believe, not unreasonably, that the patient will tell them if there's a problem. Always tell your GP about any history of illness you know of in your family. It will help him or her to build up a picture of your health and be able to decide what sort of tests you should have.

Hereditary conditions

• **Hypertension (high blood pressure)** This doesn't have any obvious symptoms but it warrants serious medical attention because it could lead to a stroke. If you have high blood pressure in your family your GP will need to check yours at least every two years.

• **Heart disease** If heart disease runs in your family you should have your cholesterol checked. You may be told to go on a special diet or given some tablets if dietary change doesn't work. You will also be advised to give up smoking.

• **Cancer of the colon** Your doctor may insist you have a colonoscopy if someone in your family has already had this disease. If you have ulcerative colitis it's especially important you have your whole bowel checked.

• **Prostate cancer** If your dad had prostate cancer let your GP know and he or she will give you rectal and blood tests to find out whether you're likely to have a problem too.

• **Chronic glaucoma** (excess pressure behind the eye). This disease runs in families and is easily spotted by an optician.

• **High cholesterol** If it's in the family, get your cholesterol checked. The doctor will know whether it needs to be monitored.

The good GP guide

Our lives are in their hands, so why do we
spend more time choosing a car than a doctor?
There are lots of excellent GPs out there so
spend time finding yourself one of the best.

Key qualities

If nothing else your GP will be well qualified. All doctors
undergo a rigorous education that includes five years at
medical school and at least four years post-graduate specialist
training as a junior doctor. Some will gain further
qualifications to become members of the Royal College of
General Practitioners. But all this training counts for nothing if
you can't get on with your doctor. Look for someone who you
can freely communicate with and who doesn't talk down to you.

Questions to ask yourself

When you next see your doctor ask yourself these
questions to see whether he or she measures up:
• Is your doctor really listening to you?
• Are you comfortable with his or her manner?
• Can you ask questions easily?
• Does your GP ask for your opinions?
• Does your doctor look at you when you're speaking?
• Does your doctor speak in jargonese or plain English?
• Does he or she explain how the practice works?
• Does your doctor offer to give you a full examination
before deciding to offer tests?
• Does your doctor use drugs sparingly and advise you
about possible side affects?
• Does he or she give you general advice on leading a
healthy life and offer to monitor your blood pressure
and weight?
• If your doctor doesn't know the answer to something
do they offer to look it up for you?

Your rights

Your doctor is required by law to inform you of your options before performing tests or starting treatment. You also have the right to expect your doctor to explain everything about your condition in simple terms, including its cause and treatment. The doctor should tell you the purpose and risks of any procedure he or she suggests. Any alternative courses of action should also be pointed out, including risks and benefits.

Specialised help

The Patient's Charter states that when your GP thinks it necessary you have the right to be referred to a consultant acceptable to you. You can choose to see a private specialist or attend a clinic in a NHS hospital. If you're admitted to hospital it will be under the care of a consultant who leads a team of doctors. If you're seen by a doctor you should also be able to see the consultant. You are entitled to a second opinion.

Private versus NHS

• If you are faced with a long wait for NHS treatment and can afford it you may consider seeing a private doctor. Among the benefits of going private are a choice of appointment times or admission dates, a choice of consultant who will perform surgery personally, a private room, and flexible visiting.
• There are drawbacks to private health care. If a GP refers you to a private practitioner you can be confident about his or her status, but if you choose one yourself you need to check qualifications and credentials.
• Private does not always mean better. Private hospitals often lack the facilities of an NHS hospital. They may not have intensive care units or specialist staff on call, and you will have to wait for the consultant to be called before any treatment can be given, which can mean a lengthy wait.
• It can be more difficult to pursue a complaint against a private practitioner because treatment is given on the basis of a contract and you may have to prove a breach of contract. You can always take up a complaint with the General Medical Council, however, as it's concerned with the conduct of both private and NHS doctors.

Complementary therapies

Complementary treatment can help conditions that are beyond the scope of conventional medicine – particularly chronic conditions, such as migraine and arthritis. Good doctors will combine conventional with complementary advice to offer the best possible health plan.

Top ten therapies

1 Osteopathy Osteopaths look for problems relating to muscles and bones. Stiffness in the shoulders from poor posture, for example, could make breathing for an asthmatic more difficult. Osteopaths will seek out "misaligned" joints, inflammation that may be causing painful pressure on nerves, and general immobility and stiffness for correction.

2 Chiropractic Chiropractors employ manipulation techniques to adjust the body's bones. These techniques maintain the correct alignment of the spine and ensure that the body's nerve supply works efficiently. By making these skeletal adjustments chiropractors can relieve pain and discomfort, increase mobility, and provide a route to better health.

3 Acupuncture Practitioners believe that sticking fine needles into specific body points stimulates the body's energy pathways, or *chi*. The conventional explanation is that the needles release the body's natural painkillers (endorphins) into the bloodstream. Acupuncture is usually used to relieve pain and to ease withdrawal from substance abuse.

4 Herbal medicine Many of the conventional remedies we take today have their roots in herbal medicine. The opium poppy, for example, is the original source of morphine. Herbalists try to find the underlying cause of illness rather than treat symptoms. They treat the body holistically and believe that herbal remedies can help the body to heal itself by restoring harmony and balance. They claim to be able to help cure a range of chronic health conditions.

5 **Homeopathy** An 18th-century German doctor, Samuel Hahnemann, developed an ancient Greek idea that certain natural substances cause symptoms that kick-start the body into self-healing. He gave his patients tiny portions of substances to enhance the body's resistance to disease. Among the illnesses modern homeopaths claim to treat are acne, asthma, colic, cystitis, eczema, heartburn, insect bites and stings, and irritable bowel syndrome.

6 **Hypnotherapy** One of the key principles of hypnotherapy is that the mind works at different levels of consciousness. During hypnosis, the conscious mind is put on standby, which allows the subconscious mind to become susceptible to suggestions from the hypnotherapist. It is often used to help people with psychological concerns or problems of addiction – notably nicotine addiction.

7 **Massage** Masseurs stroke, knead, and press muscles and tissues to help you relax mentally and physically. Gentle massage is good for releasing endorphins, while stronger massage can increase blood flow and clear the body of the toxic products of metabolism.

8 **Relaxation and visualisation** These techniques rely on the power of imagination to help you cope with stress, achieve ambitions, or even activate the self-healing process. Many doctors regard relaxation and visualisation as useful tools to aid positive thinking and reduce anxiety and depression. Practitioners believe visualisation can be used to control pain, allergies, and even immune system disorders.

9 **Aromatherapy** By using essential oils extracted from certain plants, aromatherapists claim to improve our sense of well being and alleviate headaches and nervous tension. Oils can be diluted for massaging, inhaled, or added to a bath.

10 **Reflexology** Reflexologists believe that every part of the body is mapped to the feet, and that by feeling for tender points in the feet they can detect imbalances in the body's organs. They claim that massaging tender points in the feet helps to activate the corresponding organ's healing power.

Drug treatments

Drugs are fantastic allies in the fight against illness, but only if they are taken carefully and sparingly. Pop too many pills and you may feel the benefits of the drug being countered by unpleasant side effects.

Drug awareness

There are approximately 8000 drugs available on the market with new ones appearing every week. They're designed to either cure an ailment or treat a symptom of an ailment. As drugs are powerful chemicals it's important you know what you're taking. Your doctor should explain why you need the medication, inform you of potential side effects, and tell you about food or drugs (including alcohol) that you should avoid.

What you should ask your doctor

Studies show that doctors often leave their patients in the dark when it comes to drug treatments. One way of keeping track of what you've been prescribed is by staying loyal to one pharmacist. He or she will have all your records on computer. The next time your doctor starts to fill out a prescription pad, ask him or her the following questions:

• When should I take the medication?
• How often should I take the drug and at what dosage?
• Should I avoid certain foods?
• Should I take it with food or on an empty stomach?
• What should I do if I forget to take a dose?
• What are the possible side effects?
• Can I take over-the-counter medicines with the drug?
• Is there a cheaper drug that does the same job?
• What are the trade and generic names of the drug?
• Are there any alternative treatments that do not involve drugs?

How drugs work

• Once a tablet has been swallowed it takes about an hour to be absorbed via the digestive system and arrive at the target area.

• Muscle contractions help push the drug through your oesophagus, which leads from the mouth down to the stomach, by means of peristalsis.

• In the stomach, the drug is broken down into molecules, which are absorbed through the stomach wall into blood vessels. If the drug is coated it will travel further down the digestive tract before it is broken down and passes into the bloodstream.

• The drug molecules then travel to the liver where they are broken down further before they are distributed around the body via the bloodstream.

• Only a tiny percentage of the drug actually reaches its target because the body excretes drugs as toxins.

Common generic-name drugs

1 **Nifedipine** Prescribed to treat angina and high blood pressure. Side effects: dizziness, headache, heartburn, low blood pressure, flushes, muscle weakness and cramps, palpitations, nausea, congestion, sore throat.

2 **Enalapril maleatel** Used to treat high blood pressure. Side effects: fatigue, headache, dizziness, and, less frequently, diarrhoea, nausea, impotence, ringing in the ears, cough, skin rash.

3 **Omeprazole** Suppresses gastric acid secretion in ulcer patients. Side effects: abdominal pain, constipation, diarrhoea, flatulence, nausea, vomiting, acid regurgitation, headache.

4 **Fluoroxetine** Used to treat depression and obsessive-compulsive disorders. Side effects: skin rash, fatigue, sweating and gastrointestinal complaints. It may also interfere with cognitive and motor performance.

5 **Simvastatin** Lowers cholesterol. Side effects: headache, abdominal pain, constipation, diarrhoea, flatulence, nausea.

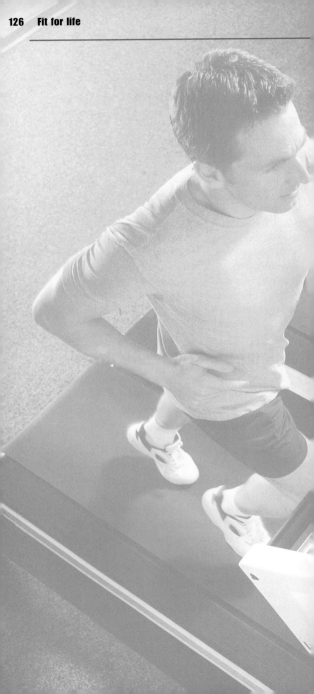

Fit for life

Why bother?

Modern lifestyles mean that we no longer
keep fit through necessity. Unfortunately,
evolution has not yet caught up with our
sedentary way of life and we need to exercise
to keep our bodies in a natural, healthy state.

The perils of inactivity

If you've had a hard day at the office, stopping off for exercise on
the way home is probably the last thing you feel like doing. But
if you don't exercise regularly your body suffers, both physically
and mentally. You are more likely to be overweight, out of
breath, and suffer from ailments ranging from muscular soreness
to stress. The fitter you are, the more fat in your body turns to
muscle and that means a stronger, leaner, more attractive you.

The endorphin high

The endorphin high is the feeling of elation many people
experience during exercise. Endorphins are opiate
proteins with pain-relieving properties found naturally in
the brain. They are released from the brain's pituitary
gland into the body during vigorous exercise and they
have similar effects on the body as morphine (another
name for endorphins is endomorphins). Morphine is a
powerful, externally-administered opiate drug, the most
important effect of which is the relief of severe and
persistent pain. Natural endorphins, therefore, can
reduce your sensitivity to pain (or have an "analgesic"
affect). Endorphins are also responsible for generating
feelings of pleasure and they can elevate your mood. It's
worth noting, however, that they don't always have a
positive effect on mood – some people may experience
negative mood changes after exercise although this is
relatively rare. The endorphin high is one explanation of
why people become addicted to exercise.

Top reasons to exercise

1 **Reduce risk of heart disease** If you never exercise you are more likely to suffer coronary heart disease or strokes. Research statistics have shown that inactive people are at double the risk of heart disease compared with those who are fit.

2 **De-stress** Sport gives your mind a break from worrying about day-to-day problems, and it's an excellent way of ridding yourself of feelings of anxiety and stress. Activities that look stressful, such as football or martial arts, often have the opposite effect.

3 **Socialise** Exercising is a great way of improving your social life. Accept your friend's invitation to join a sports club or gym or look one up in the 'phone book. Meeting up with a friend or a group of mates regularly can be a great motivation to exercise. Working out on your own, on the other hand, can sometimes be soul-destroying and there's no one to persuade you not to watch TV instead.

4 **Join a gym** Aerobic exercise, such as swimming and cycling, helps to improve general fitness levels and is especially good at improving cardiovascular fitness. Most leisure centres or gyms have classes aimed at different standards so you can choose the class that is right for you.

5 **Stay young** Exercise delays some of the effects of ageing. By doing stretching exercises, for example, you are less likely to suffer from stiff joints as you get older.

6 **Be confident** Regular exercise can give your confidence levels a real boost. Not only will you radiate a healthy glow, but you will also experience a sense of well being that other people will pick up on. And it goes without saying that women prefer their fella's flesh hard and muscular rather than fat and flabby.

7 **Stay slim** Western diets contain far too much fat. By regularly working out you can burn off the excess calories and bring down your weight.

How fit are you?

However fit you are you need to set yourself personal benchmarks before starting an exercise regime. That way you'll have the pleasure of seeing your fitness improve each week.

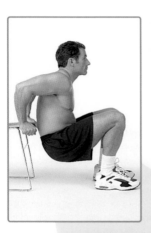

UPPER BODY STRENGTH

Chair dips Start by sitting on the edge of a chair. Holding on to the chair, lower yourself until your upper arms are parallel with the floor. Lift yourself back up level with the chair seat while keeping your back straight. If you can manage ten dips, that's a good result. Aim to build the number up over time.

LOWER BODY STRENGTH

Slow squats Stand with your feet shoulder width apart. Keeping an eye on a watch or clock, slowly bend your knees until your thighs are parallel with the floor. Then raise yourself back up as slowly as you can. If you can stretch this out for one minute, that's a good result. Aim to improve on this over a period of time.

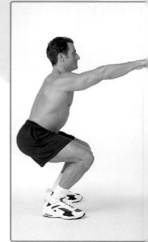

Simple fitness tests

The following easy exercises can be used as the basis for fundamental measures of fitness. Repeat these tests regularly during your exercise regime so you can keep tabs on your progress. Push your furniture to one side and spend a few minutes doing these four exercises to gauge your fitness.

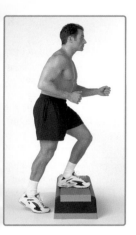

AEROBIC FITNESS

Step test Step up with one foot, then the other. Then step down with one foot, then the other. This cycle represents one count. Step for about 20 counts per minute for three minutes. Take your pulse for 15 seconds then multiply it by four. A good result is 95 beats per minute if you're in your 30s or 40s.

FLEXIBILITY

Toe touches Outstretch your left leg and fold your right leg into your body. Reach out with the left hand towards your toes – the aim is to touch your toes. Repeat on the right.

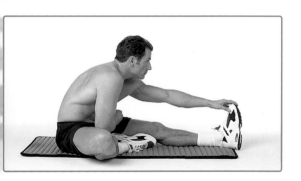

The new you

The transformation into a new, fitter you will not happen overnight. Patience and a well-planned exercise programme will determine whether you achieve your fitness goals.

Starting out

• If you haven't exercised for a long time it's important not to rush into anything too vigorous, too quickly. At best you'll soon become disenchanted and give up – and at worse you could cause yourself a long-term injury.

• Generally you should be aiming to improve your overall fitness by doing all three types of exercise – aerobic, strength training, and stretching – which, in turn, correspond to endurance, muscle tone, and flexibility.

• Some exercises will be easier for you than others depending on your physical make-up. By focusing on your strengths not only will you be fitter, but you will also have more fun.

Setting goals

Before you start exercising you should ask yourself what you want to achieve. Obviously, a would-be body builder's exercise needs differ vastly from that of a novice marathon runner. If you don't know where to begin speak to a personal trainer or the staff at your local gym. A trainer can help you to set goals and draw up a realistic exercise programme. You will also be alerted to any inefficiencies and unrealistic expectations, and informed of proper techniques and safety aspects. Start off gently – perform within your limits at first and slowly build up the intensity, duration, and frequency of exercise. Joining a decent gym or buying a good piece of home gym equipment can help motivate you to train. If you're taking up a new sport, don't shell out a fortune on kit until you're sure it's what you want to do.

Body types

There are different human body types that make some of us
more suitable for particular exercises or sports. We can't
change our basic body form and it sets natural limits to what
we can achieve. We can, however, exercise to make the best of
our strengths by building on and modifying what our genes
have determined. Whether you're an ectomorph, a
mesomorph, or an endomorph there are plenty of activities
that can bring out the best in your body.

ECTOMORPH
• Build: Tall, thin physique.
• Muscle: Limited amounts, mainly of the slow-twitch variety,
which makes it especially suitable for aerobic exercise. Slow-
twitch muscles are very resistant to fatigue. They break down
the fuel they need to contract at a slow rate and they have a
slow contraction velocity. Such muscles are typically found in
the muscles that maintain posture over prolonged periods,
notably in the back and neck.
• Tendency to fat: Ectomorphs have fast metabolic rates and a
small proportion of body fat. They will remain lean even if
they only exercise moderately.

MESOMORPH
• Build: Strong and muscular with broad-shoulders and narrow
waists; mesomorphs are society's idea of the perfect male.
• Muscle: Powerful muscles ideal for athletic pursuits.
• Tendency to fat: Their medium metabolism and small
proportion of body fat means they will remain a paragon of
male beauty as long as they exercise regularly.

ENDOMORPH
• Build: Strong and heavy physique
• Muscle: Powerful, fast-twitch muscles, which can easily
develop great strength. These muscle fibres break down the
fuel they need to contract at a fast rate and can contract
quickly and powerfully. Such muscles are typically found in the
leg muscles of sprinters.
• Tendency to fat: A slow metabolism and a large proportion
of body fat means that they will almost certainly pile on the
pounds if they don't exercise enough or eat healthy food.

Choosing your exercise

Don't let exercise be a chore. Whatever your circumstances or body type there's an activity out there that you can enjoy.

Factors to consider

• Although your body type will influence your choice of exercise (see previous page), there are other factors to consider.
• Your family life may affect your choice of exercise, and your willingness to spend money on equipment may also influence which activity or sport you pursue.
• Whatever exercise you choose, ensure it includes a mix of aerobic and strength training and stretching. Aerobic exercise promotes endurance and cardiovascular fitness, while weight lifting helps to build muscles. Stretching will help you stay flexible and will delay the onset of creaking bones.

Home or gym?

Ideally your life will be flexible enough for you to work out at the gym or home, but certain factors will force you to decide where to go to work yourself up into a sweat:

HOME
• Cheap and convenient
• 24-hour opening
• No one hogging your favourite equipment
• Radio and TV volume controlled by you
• After initial investment equipment is easy to maintain
• Equipment is always set up for your use
• Less likely to cause self-consciousness

GYM
• Equipment is up-to-date and plentiful
• Specialist advice is available from trained staff
• Atmosphere provides validation, motivation, and encouragement
• Surroundings may be more appealing, depending on status of club
• Ideal for socialising
• Bigger clubs have childcare facilities

Exercise menu

SPORT	BENEFITS	DRAWBACKS
Cycling Choose from road cycling, mountain biking, or indoor machine cycling	Good for toning leg muscles and for general cardiovascular fitness	Muscle benefits largely limited to legs; road cycling could lead to an accident
Football An energetic team game played by more and more middle-aged men	Very good aerobic exercise; sociable and exciting	High injury risk because of possible contact accidents
Golf A sport no longer confined to middle management for networking	Mild aerobic benefit; gets you outdoors; social side is good for mental health	Potential back and spine injuries; green fees can be very expensive
Racquet sports Every locality boasts at least one tennis court to get people outdoors	Vigorous aerobic and muscular exercise; competition makes it exciting	Tough on joints; need access to courts, which may be overcrowded in summer
Running Everyone was born to run – all you need are trainers	Cheap – you can run pretty much anywhere at any time	High impact activity that can cause problems in lower body joints
Swimming One of the best all-round ways of keeping fit	Combines aerobic and whole-body muscular conditioning; low impact	Requires training in basic skills and safety; ongoing cost of pool entrance

Enjoying training

If you're not motivated to train you will be tempted to give up, so it's important to set yourself realistic goals and enjoy the exercise.

Pleasure not pain

• Ask many sportsmen about motivation and they'll say that the hardest part of training is leaving the comfort of their armchair and actually getting to the gym.

• Enjoyment is the key. If you're looking forward to exercising then you'll be more likely to pull on your trainers. Training can be fun if you vary the exercise routines and make it sociable.

Seeking inspiration

• If you've decided to get fit one of your first ports of call should be your local gym or sports centre. Speak to staff about facilities and fitness classes and find out how they can help you to devise a training programme.

• Gym notice boards are worth a look as they give an idea of all the activities on offer, including sports clubs and groups you can join.

• One way to inspire yourself is to watch the valiant efforts of others. Watching the heroics of marathon runners while you stand idly by may be enough to shame you into starting your training regime.

• Magazines are another source of motivation as you can check out other people's training schedules and diets. They can also make you feel like you belong to a scene.

• Personal trainers are paid to motivate you and they will make sure your training programme is enjoyable and totally suited to your capabilities. Most personal trainers will also visit you at home if you prefer.

• Exercise with a friend. Mutual encouragement will help you when the going gets tough, and if you develop a healthy rivalry the shame of being beaten will give you another reason not to welch out of training.

Top tips for enjoyable exercise

1 **Warm up** For the first 5–10 minutes do a light aerobic activity, such as jogging. By slowly building up the heart rate you will gradually increase the oxygen flow to the muscles and prepare the body for more vigorous exercise.

2 **Stretch** After warming up spend five minutes gently stretching. It will help you extend your ranges of motion and lower the risk of injury. Be careful not to overstretch your muscles, especially those affecting the spine.

3 **Get into the habit** Make a habit of exercising because if you only train when you feel like it, your training programme will soon grind to a halt. Look through your diary and put aside two to three hours a week for exercise. Eventually it will become part of your routine.

4 **Push yourself** After two to three weeks of training you should start to work your muscles to fatigue. The only way you will build up your muscles is by doing strength exercises until your body can handle no more.

5 **Short, sharp sessions** If you're always on the go and haven't got time to train, try taking bite-size chunks of exercise. During a day, three 10-minute spells of exercise have been shown to have as much benefit as a single 30-minute session.

6 **Cool down** Spend 5–10 minutes after the exercise cooling down. It will stop your muscles from tightening and relax you mentally.

7 **Drink water** Whenever you exercise your body loses water 258 times faster than when it is at rest. If you lose just 2 percent of your body weight in fluid, your capacity for exercise will fall by 10 percent. Keep a bottle of water close by and take regular sips throughout your workout.

8 **Keep moving** Working between 75–85 percent of your maximum heart rate is ideal for improving aerobic fitness. The heart rate should stay in this range throughout the workout. Stopping suddenly can cause dizziness.

Exercise and age

As you get older your exercise needs change.
Your body may not be able to stand so much
punishment in the gym, but it's still capable
of a vast range of enjoyable exercises that will
help you to stay healthy.

Never give up

Just because your body feels a little frayed around the edges
doesn't mean you should give up on exercise. Some form of
fitness training is vital if you want to reap the benefits of good
health in your later years. The dramatic deterioration in the
health of professional footballers when they retire should
serve as a warning to us all.

When to exercise caution

If you're embarking on an exercise programme later on
in life, you should first check with your GP to see
whether you have a condition that could be aggravated
by a certain type of exercise:

Pain
Pain is a warning light, and its signals are rarely false. If
you feel pain when working out, don't try to tough it
out as you'll only increase the discomfort and pain and
aggravate any underlying injury.

Dizziness
Feeling dizzy doesn't always indicate anything serious,
but it is a warning sign associated with many illnesses,
including heart disease, strokes, and diabetes.

Chest pain
It probably doesn't mean you're about to keel over from
a heart attack, but it is worth checking out all the same.
Symptoms of a clogged artery or arteries, which can lead
to heart attacks, include difficulty breathing,
clamminess, nausea, and tingling in the neck or left arm.

What happens as you age

• **In your twenties** At this age you're in your physical peak and you may not even bother exercising. This is a mistake because you will find it harder to start later on when exercise becomes more crucial to your health.

• This is the best time to start weight training. By building up muscles now you will be in a better position to deal with the gradual reduction in muscle mass and bone density that begins in your thirties. As your body is still pumping out lots of testosterone, you will also find it easier to increase the size of your muscles at this age.

• A twenty-something body also has better recuperative powers than older models, which makes them less injury prone and more suitable to contact sports.

• **In your thirties** Your body's muscle mass, strength, aerobic capacity, and metabolic rate will start to decline. If you're still active you'll barely sense any difference. The most noticeable physical decline will probably be flexibility.

• It's prudent at this age to reduce the amount of contact and high-impact exercise you're doing. During a workout spend less time doing aerobic exercises and more time stretching.

• **In your forties** This is the period when you'll start to notice your body ageing, especially if you're inactive. It shouldn't affect your exercise regime too much, but you should shift the emphasis towards low-impact exercise to minimise the stress.

• Don't entirely abandon weight training, as you need muscle to help burn off calories and protect you from injury. Circuit training offers an ideal mix.

• Exercise helps to ward off middle-age spread, which occurs as your metabolism slows down.

• In your 40s you're also more at risk from heart disease and other serious ailments, so it's even more important to stay fit.

• **In your fifties and beyond** If you've been active all your life you'll be in a better state at this stage than a man who's always been sedentary. Bear in mind though that loss of bone mass will make you more susceptible to fractures, which may affect your future mobility. Try weight-bearing exercises where you remain on your feet, such as walking and dancing.

• At this age you're more susceptible to injury, but this varies among individuals. It's advisable to consult your GP before exercising for the first time in your fifties.

Exercise for life

If you've decided to get fit don't let your enthusiasm get the better of you by overdoing it early on. If you plan a suitable programme you're less likely to give up in the long run.

Suitability is key

For an exercise programme to be successful it should take into account your fitness, age, and lifestyle. Speak to a personal trainer or to gym staff, and make sure you update your training programme regularly.

Top tips for routine exercise

1 **Walking** This underrated activity can result in major improvements in fitness. Research has shown that if you walk briskly four or five times a week for up to 45 minutes, your blood pressure, cholesterol levels, and weight will all fall. Make walking part of your day by parking your car away from the office or walking to a sandwich shop at lunchtime. You could also try getting a dog to take you for a walk.

2 **Stair climbing** It may not be practical if you work on the 41st floor but, generally, where there's an option take the stairs rather than the lift or escalator. Underground stations, offices, and shops all offer excellent facilities.

3 **Cycling** This can be easily incorporated into your daily routine. Why not cycle to work, for instance, or at least cycle to the local shops? It's a great aerobic exercise and will leave you feeling invigorated and alert.

4 **Housework** Not only will housework help keep you in trim, but all that polishing, vacuum cleaning, and dusting will get you into your partner's good books.

5 **Sex** Regular bouts of vigorous lovemaking does wonders for the heart and helps burn off any unsightly fat.

Adjusting your exercise to your age

YOUR TWENTIES
Strength training
30 minutes three times a
week. Do three sets of
each exercise

Aerobic exercise
15–20 minutes three times
a week at 80–85 percent of
your maximum heart rate

Stretching
Five minutes during every
workout

Special concerns
Protect your joints during
contact sports

YOUR THIRTIES
Strength training
20 minutes three times a
week. Do two sets of
each exercise

Aerobic exercise
30 minutes three times a
week at 80–85 percent of
your maximum heart rate

Stretching
Five to ten minutes during
every workout

Special concerns
Stop if your body cries out
in pain

YOUR FORTIES
Strength training
20 minutes twice a week.
Do two sets of each exercise.
Circuit train for 45 minutes
once a week with lighter
weights for three circuits

Aerobic exercise
25 minutes twice a week at
60–70 percent of maximum.
Do 30 minutes of light
activity twice a week also

Stretching
Regular five–ten minutes

Stretching
Add more abdominal
exercises to offset any spread

YOUR FIFTIES PLUS
Strength training
20 minutes twice a week
and 45 minutes of circuit
training once a week using
lighter weights

Aerobic exercise
20 minutes twice a week at
60–70 percent of maximum
heart rate. Walk briskly for
30 minutes twice a week

Stretching
Regular five–ten minutes

Stretching
Avoid placing stress on the
joints and back – both areas
that are vulnerable to injury

Motivation

Why is it that on some days you can't wait to get into the gym to exercise, while on others you'd rather be at home cutting your toenails? If you can understand your motivation, you can work out an exercise programme that you'll be able to stick to.

Each to his own

We are all motivated in different ways. Some people, for example, may find that TV's Mr Motivator actually does motivate them to train, while for others the thought of showing off their muscular physique on the beach during the holidays is enough to make a commitment. Training with a friend makes exercise more pleasurable.

Common cop-outs

1 **"I've got better things to do."** Research indicates that you need only walk for 20–30 minutes three times a week to be healthy. Even if you can't find the time to join a gym, at least go for a walk during your lunch break. You won't regret it when you start feeling healthier and losing weight.

2 **"Exercise is boring."** Make sure you do an exercise you enjoy. If you have really bad memories of cross-country running at school then don't run – there's bound to be an alternative that suits you. Remember that exercise is more interesting if it's varied and done with friends.

3 **"I've been lifting weights for two months, I've put on weight, and don't feel any fitter. What's the point?"** Strength exercises aren't always ideal for those starting out. They should first concentrate on aerobic exercise, which will elevate the heart rate and help reduce weight. Stretching is a perfect exercise for beginners as it increases the level of flexibility and reduces the risk of injuries later on. Get a stretch sequence under your belt in readiness for weights.

4 **"I found the exercises too tough."** The old adage that there's no gain without pain has been responsible for a lot of injuries and abandoned training programmes. Don't push yourself too hard, especially at the start, otherwise you'll end up dreading training and give up. To benefit from exercise you only have to work up to the point where you experience tolerable discomfort.

5 **"I'd like to exercise but I need advice on what to do."** Visit your local sports centre. They should be able to provide you with some free advice about getting started. Personal trainers cost money, but they will be able to give you help specific to your needs.

6 **"I don't care what I look like, I've got a partner."** Letting yourself go once you've found a partner is a dangerous ploy in these socially mobile times. She might just trade you in for a younger, fitter, more attractive model if you can't satisfy her physical needs.

Five ways to stay motivated

1 **Have an outcome in mind** Aiming to climb a mountain, beat a personal best, or run a marathon will help you maintain your drive. Also set yourself goals in the short term as your final objective may sometimes seem too distant.

2 **Don't compare** There will always be somebody fitter than you, and that includes your younger self, so only focus on improving your present capabilities.

3 **Don't take it too seriously** Don't quit because it's not going as well as you planned. If you slacken off it doesn't matter, you can always increase your work rate in the future.

4 **Make priorities** Exercise will ultimately provide great satisfaction. When you're tempted away from exercise dwell on the benefits you'll lose out on.

5 **Have fun** Remember exercise doesn't have to be grim. Having fantastic sex, cycling down a sunny country lane, or scoring the winning goal for your team aren't chores.

Getting equipped

Cutting a dash in the gym isn't the most important aspect of training, but if you don't have the right kit you'll be less inclined to exercise if your motivation is already low.

Correct dressing

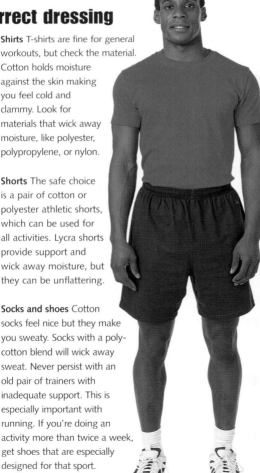

1 **Shirts** T-shirts are fine for general workouts, but check the material. Cotton holds moisture against the skin making you feel cold and clammy. Look for materials that wick away moisture, like polyester, polypropylene, or nylon.

2 **Shorts** The safe choice is a pair of cotton or polyester athletic shorts, which can be used for all activities. Lycra shorts provide support and wick away moisture, but they can be unflattering.

3 **Socks and shoes** Cotton socks feel nice but they make you sweaty. Socks with a poly-cotton blend will wick away sweat. Never persist with an old pair of trainers with inadequate support. This is especially important with running. If you're doing an activity more than twice a week, get shoes that are especially designed for that sport.

Setting up a home gym

If you're serious about being fit installing a home gym is a great idea, as long as you consider the following points:

• Some careful negotiations with your partner may be in order if you're about to convert the spare room into your own personal gym.

• Devise a plan for moving out the jumble and empty boxes.

• If the room hasn't been used for a while give it a lick of paint and throw in a few pot plants, otherwise you won't feel like going in there.

• Make sure the room can be heated in the winter and cooled in the summer.

• Measure your floor area before buying bulky exercise machines to make sure everything fits.

• Check the ceiling height. It can constrict the use of some items of equipment. This is especially important in the case of a budding trampolinist.

Top tips for buying trainers

1 **Check sizes** Don't trust the sizes written on the side of the boxes – shoes can vary from box to box. For this reason don't go for mail order trainers unless there's a generous returns policy.

2 **Make sure the shoes fit** There should be about 1cm ($\frac{1}{2}$in) of breathing space between the toes and the tip of the shoe; the ball of the foot should fit comfortably into the shoe's widest point; and the heel should fit snugly without slipping. Ignore the advice of the sales person who tells you that the shoes will probably stretch – if the shoes don't fit when you're in the shop, don't buy them.

3 **Try both** Try on both shoes as sometimes one foot may be smaller than the other. Also, make sure that the shoes in the pair are the same size.

4 **Leave your shoe shopping until last** Your feet swell by as much as 5 percent during the day, so buying when they're full size should ensure that the shoes are not too tight.

Warming up

Warming up may seem trivial alongside your Herculean efforts in the weights room, but if you skip it you'll compromise your performance and, worse, risk injury.

Warm and stretch

• There are two phases to a warm up. First, spend 5–10 minutes doing a light activity, such as jogging, or one of the exercises listed opposite. This phase helps raise body temperature, which makes your ligaments, muscles, and tendons more pliable.

• Gentle exercise also helps increase the blood flow to your muscles. This means the muscles benefit from more nutrients and oxygen, which results in more power and endurance.

• Always follow the warm up with phase two: 5–10 minutes of stretching exercises.

Top tips for warming up

1 **Warm the muscles** Don't stretch your muscles when they're cold. Make sure the gentle warm up comes first or you'll end up pulling a muscle before you've even started.

2 **Pace it** Warm up until you have broken into a light sweat. You don't want to finish the warm up out of breath. Save your energy for the main event.

3 **Exercise all muscle groups** When stretching be sure to exercise as many muscle groups as possible and hold each stretch for 30 seconds. See pages 176–177 for examples of good stretching exercises.

4 **Cool down** If you warm up half-heartedly, you probably skip or skimp on the cool down as well. The cool down helps to restore energy to muscles, it contributes to the removal of lactic acid, and it prevents blood from rushing to your extremities and making you dizzy.

Jogging on the spot Make exaggerated running motions with your upper arms while you jog gently. Alternatively, you can swing your arms round in circles. Make sure that your heels make contact with the floor on each step.

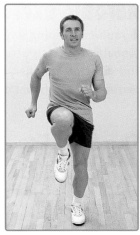

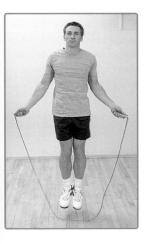

Skipping A more vigorous alternative to jogging that's good for the muscles: jump with both feet together, keeping movements small and close to the floor.

Cycling If you can cycle to your gym it's ideal – if not use an exercise bike. Pedal with enough speed or resistance to make you draw deep breaths. Alternatively, try stair stepping. Step up and down a stair or aerobic step one foot after another. Every minute swap your lead foot. You might use a stepping machine at the gym for the same purpose. Five to ten minutes will be enough to get the blood flowing.

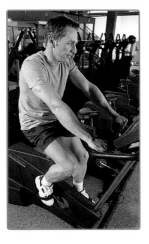

Aerobic exercise

If you're not doing any aerobic exercise you're probably overweight and your heart, lungs, and muscles are likely to be under-performing. So, what are you waiting for?

The benefits

Aerobic exercise forces the heart and lungs to work harder, which means a more efficient delivery of oxygen and nutrients to your body. The benefits are a faster metabolism, greater endurance, and protection against heart disease among other ailments.

Work that body

To become fit you must work hard, but not too hard. The training zone below shows the rate at which your heart should be beating to gain maximum benefit from aerobic exercise. Aim towards the bottom of the band.

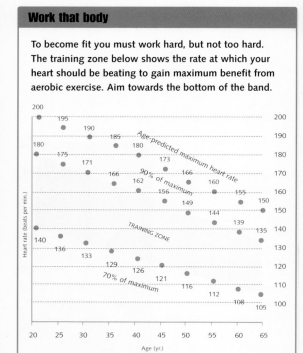

What, how, and when?

• For aerobic exercise to be of benefit your heart should be beating at around 70 percent of the age-predicted maximum (see chart, below left).

• Measure your pulse by placing two fingers on the thumb-side artery on the inside of your wrist. Count the number of beats for 15 seconds. Multiply by four to get your heart rate.

• You should exercise aerobically three times a week with a day's rest in between sessions. The rest day gives your body time to repair the microscopic damage done to your muscles.

• As aerobic activity is sustained, workouts should only be 20–30 minutes long.

• The chart below shows how many calories are burned during different activities according to how long you spend at them.

Expending calories				
ACTIVITY	15 min	30 min	45 min	60 min
Cycling				
20km/h (12 1/2 mile/h)	142	283	425	566
30km/h (18 1/2 mile/h)	213	425	638	850
Rowing	104	208	310	415
Running				
5-min. km (8-min. mile)	183	365	548	731
4-min. km (6-min. mile)	223	446	670	893
Swimming				
33m (110ft)/min	124	248	371	497
45m (150ft)/min	131	261	392	523
Circuit training	189	378	576	756
Cross-country skiing	146	291	437	583

Strength training

You don't have to be a bull-necked body builder to benefit from lifting weights. Strong, powerful muscles not only make you look and feel great, they protect you against injury.

The benefits

• A good weight training programme should lead to a flatter abdomen, bigger chest, stronger-looking arms and better-looking legs.
• You should also feel like a strongman around the home as bigger muscles make everyday household and decorating tasks easier to perform.
• The advantages don't end there. Muscle tissue requires greater amounts of energy to sustain it than fat tissue, so weight lifting will help you shed any excess pounds.

The right technique

• To ensure you have a sound weight lifting technique, consult a trainer at your local gym or in private before you begin. If you aren't lifting properly a serious injury can easily result.
• Before starting an exercise complete the movement without the weights first to make sure you are in the correct position.
• It's important that you don't lift too quickly otherwise you'll put undue stress on your muscles and tendons. Lifting slowly also ensures that momentum doesn't give you a helping hand.
• Each completed lift should take around six seconds – two seconds up and four seconds down.
• Contrary to what you may have been led to believe, the down part of the lift (known as eccentric or negative movement) actually builds muscles 20 percent faster than the up part of the movement (known as concentric or positive movement).

Top tips for improving strength

1 **Load up** The weight for any exercise should be enough to cause muscle fatigue after 8–12 lifts.

2 **Go steady** If you're new to weight training, start with weights that feel fairly light to you for the first 2–3 weeks. You should be able to do 12 repetitions (reps) without feeling too much strain. After three weeks your body should be ready to take on bigger loads. Increase the weight until eight reps feels OK but 12 feels hard. When you're doing 12 reps without a problem then increase the weight further, but not by more than 5 percent at a time.

3 **Rest** Give your muscles a chance to recover between exercises by resting for 90 seconds after a set of reps.

4 **Target groups of muscles** The body's hundreds of different muscles are grouped into seven main sets. By targeting particular sets of muscles when you train you should be able to give yourself a full-body workout by doing as few as seven different exercises.

Your strength programme

• Regular weight training improves muscle strength, size, and endurance. A tailored programme, devised with the help of a professional trainer, allows you to specifically train for improvements in each of these areas.
• By changing one of four elements – the amount of resistance, the number of repetition (reps), the number of sets, or the amount of rest time – you can determine which goal you will achieve in what order.
• The table here shows you how you can fine-tune your training programme to achieve positive changes in the endurance capacity, strength, and size of your muscles:

Goal	Resistance	Reps	Sets	Rest
Strength	Heavy	3–8	3–5	2–5min
Size	Moderate	8–12	3–5	60–90sec
Endurance	Light	12–20	2–3	15–30sec

Endurance training

By setting yourself a long-term endurance challenge, such as a marathon or triathlon, you could take your fitness to a higher plane.

Getting ready

• If you already have a good level of fitness and you want to move your training up a gear, an endurance event could provide the impetus you need.

• Aim to complete your chosen endurance event in a set period of time. Knowing that you must train consistently to achieve your goal will make you less inclined to skip training.

• The following cycling, running, and swimming schedules show that with dedication you can achieve your goals relatively quickly. The cycling and running schedules are self-explanatory. The aim of the swimming plan is to do the 100m (30ft) freestyle event as strongly and as quickly as possible.

Cycling the metric century schedule

The training to cycle 100km (62 miles) in one day includes a mixture of speeds and distances to build endurance.

Week	Mon	Tues	Wed	Thur	Fri	Sat	Sun	Total km
1	10	16	19	off	16	48	14	123
2	11	18	21	off	18	55	16	158
3	13	21	24	off	21	61	18	172
4	13	22	27	off	22	67	21	172
5	13	22	27	off	16	8	100	186

Easy   Steady   Brisk   Century day

Running a half-marathon

Week 1	If you're running 5km (3 miles) three times a week, add another 5km run on a fourth day
Week 2	Make one of your runs 6km ($3^1/_2$ miles) long. Take a day off before and after the longest run
Week 3	Add a second run of 6km, alternating the 5km with the 6km days: 6–5–6–5
Week 4	Run 6km on three days and 8km (5 miles) on the other. Take a day off either side of the longest run.
Week 5	Add another 8km run and make your longest distance day 10km (6 miles): 10-6-8-8.
Week 6	Keep running the 6s and 8s, but increase the 10km run to 13km (8 miles).
Week 7	Boost your 13km run to 16km (10 miles), which is two-thirds of the half-marathon distance. Your schedule is now: 16–6–6–8.
Week 8	Reduce training: run the same as in week 3 and take the day before the race off.

Swimming 100 metres (30ft)

MONDAYS AND WEDNESDAYS

Swim 1500–2000m (450–600ft) in segments of, say, 100 or 500m (30 or 150ft), and rest for 30 seconds after each set. You should start by swimming smaller segments, for example, 15 times 100m, and increase this to three sets of 500m. Swim at 70 percent of your capability.

TUESDAYS AND THURSDAYS

Do the same as on Mondays and Wednesdays, but work at 80 percent of your maximum effort. Cut the rest period after each set to 15 seconds.

FRIDAYS

On this day, switch into overdrive. Swim four segments of 100m at 90 percent of your maximum effort. Don't rest between segments, but keep swimming for 50m (15ft) at 60 percent of maximum effort.

The office workout

Just because you're stuck at work all day doesn't mean you have to stop exercising. With this indoor workout you don't even have to loosen your tie.

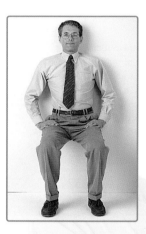

WALL SITS

Stand with your back against the wall and slide down the wall until your knees bend at right angles. To build up your legs hold this position for 5–10 seconds before sliding back up into a standing position.

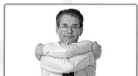

SHOULDER HUGS

Shoulder hugs are very good for relieving shoulder stress – typically suffered by desk-bound office workers who use a computer much of the time. Cross both arms over your chest, reaching back for each shoulder blade with your hands.

SEATED LEG LIFTS

You can do this simple leg-strengthening exercise without even getting up from your chair. Sit up in your chair with both legs extended and slowly raise both feet keeping your legs straight. Hold for 5 seconds and then lower your feet back down. Repeat.

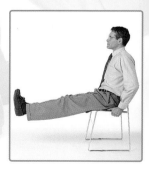

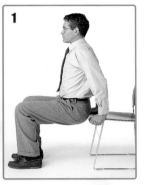 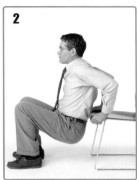

CHAIR DIPS (upper body)

1 Sit on the edge of a chair and carefully push yourself away from the edge using your hands to support yourself.

2 Lower yourself until your arms are parallel with the floor, then lift yourself back up. Repeat 8–12 times daily.

TWISTS (chest and abs)

Sit with your arms up and twist your torso from left to right. Hold for 2 seconds and repeat 3 times on each side.

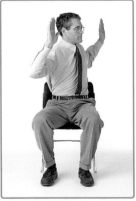

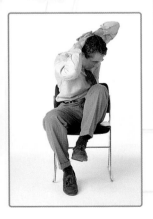

KNEE TOUCHES (abs)

Link your hands behind your head. Lift your left knee and bend your right elbow down towards it. Repeat on both sides.

Cross-training

Cross-training not only relieves the monotony of doing the same exercise over and over again, it also makes you an all-round fitter, stronger person.

The benefits

• Cross training involves mixing different types of exercise. The key benefit is that you exercise a broader range of muscles than you would if you concentrated on one activity. If you run or cycle as well as practising strength exercises, you're ensuring that your aerobic fitness isn't neglected.

• At one time fitness trainers believed that you shouldn't combine strength and aerobic exercises as you would end up doing neither very well. This has now been discredited – even serious athletes training for a specific sport realise that combining the two helps fend off boredom, reduces the risk of repetitive injury, and increases general fitness.

• Cross-training is not as technical or time-consuming as it sounds. If you're cycling to work one day and digging over the garden the next then you're already doing it.

• The most extreme form of cross-training is the triathlon. It's a combination of three long-distance events – swimming, cycling, and running – and in terms of training it requires a lot of dedication.

Mixing and matching

To achieve a good level of general fitness you should be looking to combine diverse forms of exercise. That way each activity will provide a benefit that the others are missing. To achieve a balance, bear these principles in mind:

• Mix repetitive exercises, such as running, with skilled ones, like football.

• Be kind to your joints by combining hard-impact sports, such as running or tennis, with low-impact ones, like swimming, cycling or rowing.

• Combine exercises aimed at the upper and lower body to improve your entire physique, not just your legs or torso.

Resting

• One of the most important aspects of training is rest. In fact, your muscles actually grow while you're resting and recovering. During strenuous exercise the muscle breaks down and becomes weaker. It is only by resting that muscles can be built up and made stronger.

• If you do too much training you may not give your muscles enough time to recover. The result will be pain, fatigue, loss of motivation and, if you really overdo it, injury.

• Over-reaching usually occurs at the start of a training programme when you're not used to exercise, or when you push yourself too hard in an activity.

• Always programme rest intervals into your fitness schedule.

Top tips for getting enough rest

1 **Begin gently** Proceed with care, especially at the start of an exercise programme. Your muscles won't be used to the exercise and they'll be sore even if you're not overdoing it. Start by doing less than you know you can. Then gradually increase the amount of exercise by about 10 percent per week until the post-exercise aches recede.

2 **Rest during the workout** Give your muscles a chance to recover by having rests during your programme. Giving muscles a brief respite during exercises allows them to work for longer during a session. This is particularly pertinent advice for those lifting weights.

3 **Split your routine** Give your muscles an extra day's leave after particularly strenuous workouts. This doesn't mean you have to be inactive, however, because on the next day you can exercise another set of muscles. Weight lifters call these exercises "split routines" whereby upper body exercises are alternated with lower body routines.

4 **Active rest** During your rest day you may benefit from a light activity, such as walking or cycling. Active rest may reduce soreness and help to flush out the waste products from muscles that make them function less efficiently.

Avoiding injury

You might have a personal trainer and the smartest kit, but it counts for nothing if you're injured. Find out how to avoid injury now and it could save you a lot of pain in the future.

Getting ready

• Many sports injuries are preventable and are usually caused by lack of preparation. Always make sure you're properly warmed up and are wearing appropriate shoes and clothing.
• Use the equipment correctly – ignoring the instruction manual or chart could have serious consequences.
• If you feel persistent pain while exercising call the whole session off as it could be a symptom of something serious.

Top tips for problem prevention

1 **Warming up** Warming up before your main exercise makes your muscles more pliable and less likely to tear. It also helps to lubricate the joints and it improves the muscles' ability to convert oxygen to energy at a cellular level.

2 **Stretching** Spend five minutes stretching your muscles after your initial warm up. It opens up the ranges of movement and, again, helps prevent injury.

3 **Use safety gear** Examples are weight belts and gloves and cycling helmets. If you haven't used safety gear until now and you've remained injury-free, then you've been lucky.

4 **Be informed** You can learn a lot from books and magazines, but it's also worth getting expert help and advice. Gym staff or personal trainers should advise you about kit, show you how to use exercise equipment properly, and devise a programme that doesn't put too much strain on your body.

5 **Pay attention to pain** You feel pain for a reason. It's not there to prove how tough you are when you ignore it.

When to see your doctor

It's likely that we'll all be struck down by injury at some point. Don't hesitate to see your GP if you have an inexplicable pain or discomfort:
- **Head** A feeling of disorientation or loss of consciousness following a blow on the head are signs of concussion. A blow may also cause dizziness, confusion, headache, nausea, weakness, or fatigue.
- **Shoulders** If you're in agony, go straight to casualty as a dislocation is likely.
- **Elbows** A feeling of tenderness may indicate bursitis (see p.80), and a persistent numbing or tingling sensation in your elbow could be a symptom of nerve damage.
- **Back** Pain that radiates down the back of the lower limbs or is accompanied by numbness or pins and needles is likely to indicate pressure on a spinal nerve.
- **Knees** If you can't extend or flex your knee or it locks, there may be a loose piece of cartilage in the joint.

Easing injury pain yourself

Sore muscles are caused by inflammation, which leads to swelling and pressure. You can soothe the pain by using the RICE method: Rest, Ice, Compression, and Elevation:

- **Rest** the injured muscle to give the tissue a chance to mend. Avoid unnecessary movements.

- **Ice** should be applied – but not directly on the skin – to constrict blood vessels and numb the pain. Don't use it for more than 20 minutes or you'll risk frost bite.

- **Compress** the area around the affected muscle by wrapping it with a bandage. This has the effect of squeezing the blood vessels and reducing the swelling.

- **Elevate** the sore muscle so it's above the heart for about 20 minutes. This will facilitate the flow of fluid out of the muscle while reducing the amount of blood that flows in.

Sports therapies

Sports massage and other alternative therapies used to be considered an indulgence in sports circles, but now their benefits have become more widely recognised.

Key practices

• Sports masseurs can help prevent injury and speed up the repair of damaged tissues by relaxing the muscles and flushing out waste products.

• Osteopaths treat problems in the muscles, joints, and bones that may be causing pain elsewhere. For example, an imbalance in the pelvis caused by a fall off a horse might cause lower back pain. Osteopaths use massage, muscle stretching, and articulation and manipulation of joints to loosen and relax muscles and free up stiff joints.

• Chiropractors track down skeletal misalignments, especially in the spine. They believe these problems cause inflammation and pressure that can lead to pain and illness in other parts of the body. Sports injuries are common causes of such problems. The chiropractor might use massage to loosen stiff muscles before moving to manipulation techniques. Manipulation usually involves sharp thrusting motions on affected joints.

• Physiotherapists treat sports injuries with exercises (passive or active), massage, heat or cold treatments, water treatments, or the application of electrical currents.

• Sports nutritionists help you make the most of exercise by advising you on how to get the right fuel – Arsene Wenger insisted that his players replaced their hamburger meals with light pasta salads. We all have slightly different nutritional needs but the healthy eating general rules apply (see p.12–21). Certain sports, however, require a different approach so if you're taking your sport seriously and aren't too sure about your diet, a sports nutritionist will direct you towards the most appropriate food for your type of exercise.

Self-massage

Sports massage, physiotherapy, chiropractic, and osteopathy are popular treatments for tired or injured tissues, all of which may incorporate soft tissue massage as part of the treatment. While a professional massage is best, you can do much to help yourself. These examples show you how:

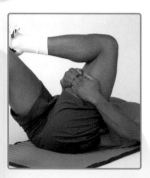

HAMSTRINGS

Sit against a wall and draw one leg up. Knead and squeeze the back of this leg before lying flat with your right knee bent and your right foot flat on the floor. Rest your left ankle on your right knee and clasp your left leg with your hands. Slide it towards your bottom.

NECK AND SHOULDERS

With your right hand press, knead, and squeeze the thick muscle behind your right shoulder. Tilt your head away from your hand while applying downward pressure towards the shoulder to stretch out the muscle. Repeat on the left side.

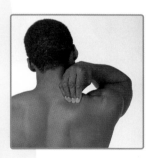

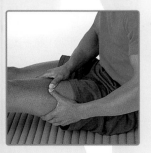

THIGHS

Use both hands to knead and squeeze the muscles at the top of a leg. Then place one hand on either side of the thigh so the thumbs meet on the top of the leg and press firmly down while pushing towards the knee. Repeat on both thighs.

Pain–free training

By practising good training techniques you should be able to avoid injuries involving speed, balance, high-impact movement, or heavy weight lifting.

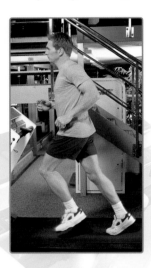

1 Running is a high-impact activity that can cause stress on muscles, tendons, and joints. This is especially true if the exercise is carried out on tarmac in poor training shoes. To minimise the injury risks, wear proper running shoes (*see p.144*), take short steps to avoid over-stretching, run on soft, even surfaces, such as a treadmill or a grass track, and adopt a relaxed running style to prevent posture strain.

2 Road cyclists are always prone to accidents so wear a helmet. Choose a helmet made by a reputable company and get it properly fitted in a cycle shop. Cycling can also be hard on backs and knees. To avoid knee injury, don't strain against the pedals in higher gears and make sure the seat's at the right height. If your back's hurting, get a mechanic to check your riding position.

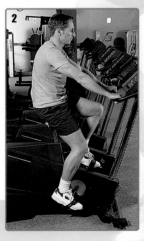

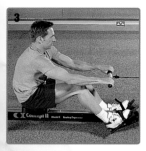

3 You're likely to strain back muscles when rowing if your movement isn't smooth and steady. To avoid strain, pull the handle towards your torso with your arms.

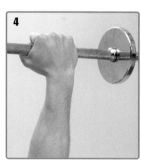

4 When weight lifting, keep joints loose and don't lock elbows or knees to avoid undue stress. Breathe out when lifting and breathe in when returning to the starting position to avoid dizziness or black-outs.

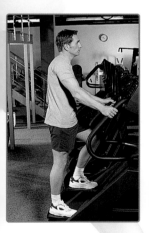

5 To avoid pressure on the neck and back during stepping or stair climbing always maintain an upward stance. Remain flat-footed as stepping on your toes puts pressure on the balls of the feet, and loose laces will help improve blood circulation.

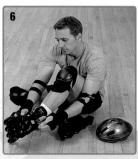

6 Accidents will happen, so get padded up, especially around the wrists. Lessons will teach you how to brake, stride, and fall.

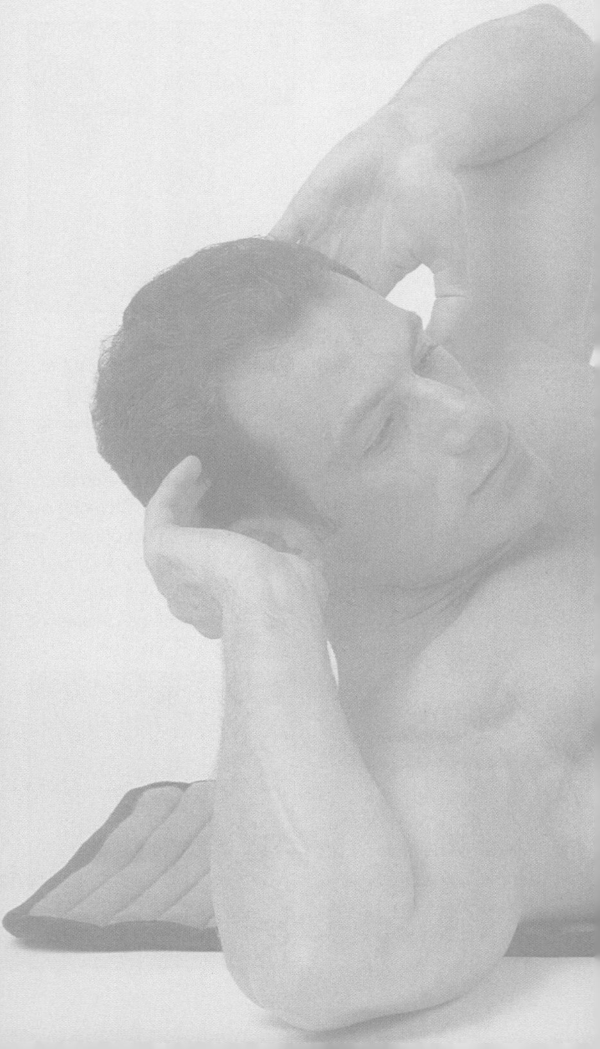

Full body exercises

Thighs and calves
Chest and shoulders
Back and biceps
Shoulder tops and triceps
Abdominals
Upper leg stretches
Hip and groin stretches
Hamstrings and calves
Back stretches
Side and chest stretches

Thighs and calves

Strengthen the quadricep (front of thigh),
hamstring (back of thigh), and calf muscles.

Squats

Squatting down and up again in a vertical position is good for
the thighs and the lower back. If you're a beginner don't worry
about using the barbell at first, but you'll only start really
strengthening muscles when you begin loading on the weights.

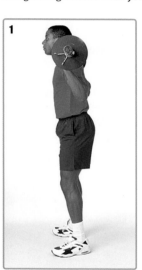
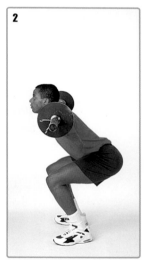

SETS 3–5
REPS 18–22

1 Stand up straight with your feet placed shoulder-width
apart. Hold a barbell across the shoulders with your palms
facing forward.

2 Lean forward slightly then bend your knees until your thighs
are parallel to the floor. Then slowly rise to the starting
position, keeping your feet flat on the floor. It's very
important to keep your back straight and well-supported
throughout the squats to prevent damage to the lower back.

Heel raises

Using your toes to lift your body weight while holding dumbbells helps to strengthen your calf muscles and foot arches.

SETS	3–5
REPS	15–25

1 Find a platform at least 7.5–10cm (3–4in) high, such as the bottom step of the stairs. Use the same platform for the calf stretches (see p.181), and ensure that you warm up your calves before using the weights.

2 Hold a dumbbell in each hand with your palms facing your legs, and position your heels so they hang over the edge of the step.

3 With the balls of your feet taking the weight of your body, lower your feet so your heels are below the level of the platform. Now raise yourself back up until your feet return to their original position.

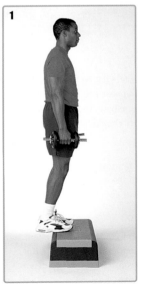

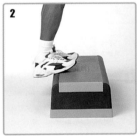

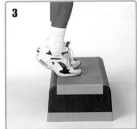

Chest and shoulders

Use these exercises to bulk up your pectoral (chest) muscles and those of your shoulders.

Dumbbell flies

This is the sort of exercise that really expands your chest muscles and benefits your upper arms. Start with moderate weights and increase them gradually as you get stronger.

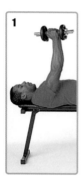
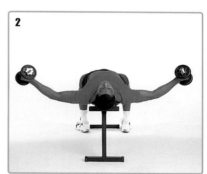

SETS	3–5
REPS	18–22

1 Lie back on a bench with your feet flat on the floor. Hold the dumbbells one in each hand over your chest with your palms facing one another. Your elbows should be slightly bent, not locked, and your back should be pressed as flat as possible against the bench.

2 Slowly lower your arms away from your body until they are outstretched and level with the chest. Your wrists should be firm and your elbows bent at about 45° throughout the exercise.

3 Slowly raise your arms back up to their starting position and then repeat the movement. Concentrate on making the chest muscles do all the work, otherwise the shoulders will take the strain and they are liable to get injured.

Alternating dumbbell press

This is a very good exercise for building up muscles in your
shoulders, including those that support your arms for lifting.

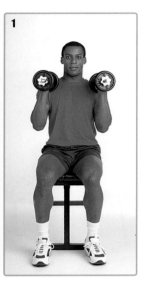 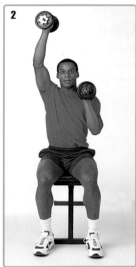

SETS 3–5
REPS 18–22

1 Sit with your legs approximately hip-width apart and your
feet flat on the floor. Sit up straight and hold a dumbbell in
each hand. Bend your elbows upwards so that you're
grasping the dumbbells at shoulder level with your palms
facing one another.

2 Lean slightly forwards and begin to lift the left dumbbell
above your head. Make sure your back is straight and well-
supported at all times to avoid straining it. Keep lifting until
your arm is straight – but don't allow your elbow to lock
straight at any time.

3 Lower the weight slowly until it has returned to the start
position, and then slowly lift the right dumbbell in the same
way. Repeat, alternating between arms.

Back and biceps

A strong back is vital for gaining strength and for lifting weights with your arms safely.

One-arm dumbbell rows

This is a good exercise for the back muscles, but you must practice good technique to avoid damage. The important thing to remember is to avoid arching your back, even when you tire.

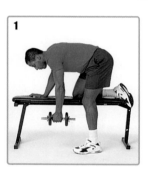 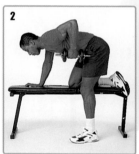

SETS 3–5
REPS 8–12

1   Put your right hand and right knee on a bench and put your other foot on the floor. Grab the dumbbell with your left hand, straighten your back, and point your head to the floor. Lower your left hand towards the floor without locking the elbow.

2   With a straight back pull up the dumbbell towards your torso. Keep pulling it upwards until your left elbow is pointing towards the ceiling and your hand is level with your lower chest muscles.

3   To gain maximum benefit from the downward movement, lower the dumbbell very slowly until you are back in the starting position. This "negative" movement is up to 20 percent more effective at building muscle than the positive upward movement, but only if you let your muscle take the strain rather than gravity or momentum. Repeat on each side.

Concentration curls

This exercise is great for building up your biceps, and excellent training if you're warming up for an arm wrestling bout in the pub.

SETS 3–5
REPS 8–12

1 Sit with your feet flat on the floor and your chest relaxed and shoulders wide apart. Extend your right arm between your legs and grab the dumbbell in your right hand with your palm facing out. To steady yourself place your left hand on your left knee.

2 Raise the dumbbell up towards your chest in an arc so that the palm eventually faces in. Stop lifting when you reach your shoulder. Your body is supported by your left hand on top of the left knee. Slowly lower the dumbbell to its starting position and then start over again, changing arms after a set of repetitions.

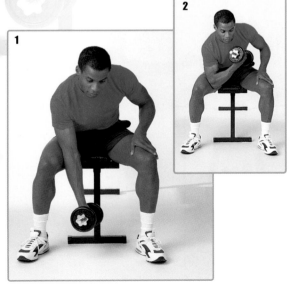

Shoulder tops and triceps

Strengthen the tops of your shoulders, the sides of your torso, and the triceps at the backs of your upper arms.

Dumbbell raises

You'll notice yourself tiring quickly at first, but you'll soon gain strength. The lifting should be slow and controlled, and the raised dumbbells should be no higher than your shoulders.

SETS 3–5
REPS 18–24

1   Stand with your feet shoulder-width apart and hold the dumbbells down by your side with your palms facing into your body. Force your shoulders back and your chest forward, and make your back as straight as a rod.

2   Raise your arms outwards and slightly forwards keeping your elbows slightly bent. Gently lower them and repeat the movement. Avoid lifting the weights too high.

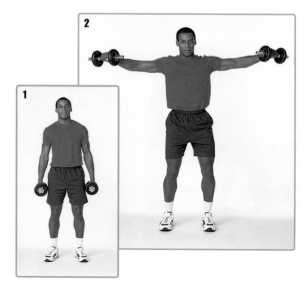

Seated triceps press

This exercise strengthens the rear shoulder muscles and backs of the upper arms. Make sure you include it in your programme as these muscles often get neglected in workouts.

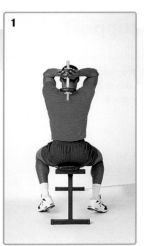 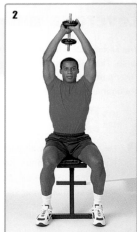

SETS 3–5
REPS 18–22

1 Sit on a bench and hold the dumbbell vertically behind your head. Grip the uppermost weight and hold it firmly with your fingers interlacing or overlapping to ensure the dumbbell doesn't slip. The elbow should be pointing up, and your arm should be near to your head.

2 Keeping your back straight, slowly life the weight towards the ceiling by extending your arm. Stop when your arm is straight but don't allow your elbow to lock. To complete the movement lower the dumbbells back down by slowly bending your elbow. Repeat sets of repetitions using each arm in turn.

3 To prevent the dumbbell from slipping, make sure the weights are screwed on securely and that you have a firm grip on the dumbbell at all times.

Abdominals

The abdominal muscles are central to many of the body's movements, so a regular workout will make you stronger all over.

Leverage and support

The abdominal muscles (abs) are at the front and sides of the torso. They provide the leverage you need to exert muscles in other parts of the body. The back also depends on the abdominal muscles to support the spine.

SETS 3–5
REPS 9–12

1   Lie on your back with your elbows to the sides and your hands by your temples. Raise your head off the floor and keep your chin clear of your chest. Your legs should be slightly apart and your knees should be at 45 degrees with both feet in contact 15cm (6in) from your buttocks.

2   Curl your torso up towards your knees, raising your shoulders off the ground. Hold the position for a second, lower to the floor again, and repeat without pausing.

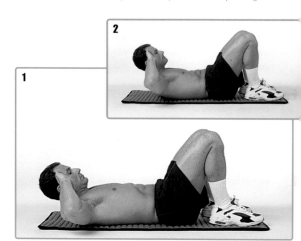

Lying toe reach

Unfortunately, abdominal exercises alone won't get rid of your flab. You may have well-toned abdominals but if you don't do aerobic fat-burning exercise like this toe reach, they'll be hidden from view.

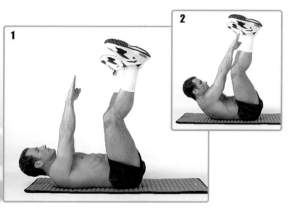

SETS 2–3
REPS 5–10

1 As with all abdominal exercises this crunch should be performed on a mat to prevent your back from being hurt. You must strive to keep your lower back in contact with the mat at all times (this is more difficult when you're raising your legs off the floor). It's easy to forget this as you become tired, and the result may be a lower back strain.

2 Lie down on your back and extend your legs upwards and outwards in a "V" shape. Your legs should be bent at the knee and the joints should be loose. In this position point your hands at the ceiling and place the palm of one hand over the back of the other.

3 Slowly curl your shoulder blades away from the mat and reach out towards the right foot with your hands. Hold for a second and then gently lower yourself back down keeping your abs contracted. Now stretch your hands towards your left foot and repeat.

Upper leg stretches

You may have bulging muscles, but if they're not flexible because you don't stretch you'll risk being the biggest stiff in the gym.

Quadriceps

Thighs are heavily-used muscles and this exercise enables them to stretch even further for difficult tennis shots and ambitious new sex positions. Having flexible thighs will also help open your stride for running and minimise the risk of pulling the often-injured quadricep muscles at the front of the thigh.

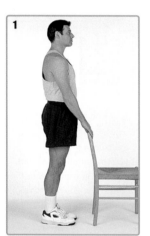
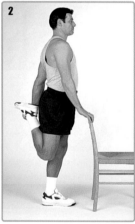

REPS **1–2**
TIME **30 secs**

1 Using a chair or the wall for support stand up straight with your feet roughly shoulder-width apart.

2 Bend your right knee behind you and grab your right foot with your left hand, while holding the chair for support. Keep your left foot slightly bent to keep stress off the knee. Gradually pull your right leg up until it touches your buttocks. Hold for 30 seconds and then repeat with the other leg.

Hips and thighs

With stretching, as with weight lifting, you should be targeting whole groups of muscles, such as those in the hips and thighs. With a minimum number of exercises you'll then be making sure that every muscle in the body is flexed. It doesn't take long either. A combination of exercises that will stretch all your muscles can be completed in 5–10 minutes just prior to your main workout.

REPS 1–2
TIME 30 secs

1 Place your left foot on a bench, the third step of a flight of stairs, or another object of a similar height. With the ball of your foot on the step, keep your right foot flat on the floor and bend your knee slightly so that your right leg is ready to absorb any excess pressure.

2 Put your hands on your hips and lean forwards into your left leg. While keeping your torso dead straight push your hips forward, but not so far that they cross the line beyond the toes of your left foot. Push until you feel the stretch in your hip and top of the thigh. Hold this position for 30 seconds and then repeat the same exercise on the other side.

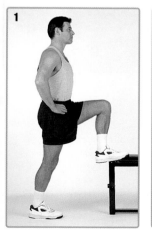

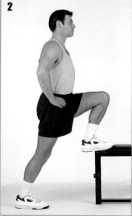

Hip and groin stretches

By stretching the muscles around the hips you are mobilising pelvic joints and improving the flexibility of the muscles close by.

Warm up first

Before you start any stretching exercise you should make sure you're warmed up first. Ideally stretching should be performed between your initial warm up and your main workout. A few minutes of light activity will make your muscles more pliable, allowing them to stretch further without injury.

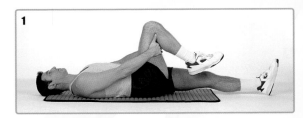

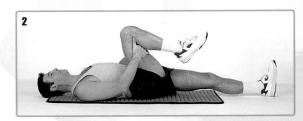

REPS **1–2**
TIME **30 SECS**

1 Get into the starting position for this exercise by lying on your back with your legs extended and grab your right leg. Interlock your fingers behind the right thigh.

2 Pull your right knee slowly towards your chest and hold for 30 seconds. Return your leg back to its original position and repeat with the left leg.

REPS 1–2
TIME 30 secs

1 Sit up straight and bring your feet together so you're perched like a frog with your knees up in the air.

2 Gently press your knees down towards the floor keeping your feet together. Hold this position for 30 seconds and repeat to loosen up the groin area.

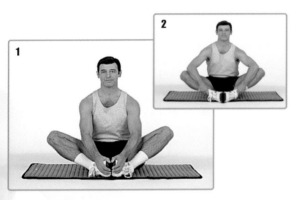

Stretching limits

• The safest form of stretching and the one most suitable for general fitness is known as static fitness. This involves slow stretching exercises that use gravity and weight to apply only a limited amount of force to push muscles just beyond their usual range of movement. All the exercises featured in this section *(p.176–185)* are static.

• For advanced stretching techniques you should consult a trainer. He or she will introduce you to dynamic, ballistic, or proprioceptive neuro-muscular facilitation (PNF) stretching.

• Dynamic stretching involves a bouncing move in which you "power" the muscle into an extended range of motion. It's best done on muscles that are already conditioned and are about to be subjected to sudden, forceful movement.

• Ballistic stretching is one step up from dynamic – it's simply quicker and more strenuous.

• With PNF stretching, a partner holds you while you isometrically contract muscles.

Hamstrings and calves

Hamstrings and calf muscles are very easily
pulled, and calves tend to cramp if unstretched.

How long to hold?

Researchers have found that 30 seconds is the most beneficial
time to hold a hamstring stretch. A 15-second stretch is little
better than doing nothing, while holding for more than
60 seconds offers no more benefits than holding for 30.

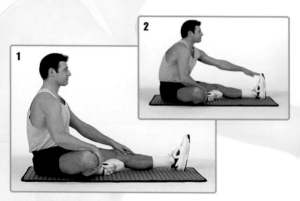

REPS	1–2
TIME	30 SECS

1 Sit with your leg straight out in front of you and bend the
right knee so your right foot is resting against your left thigh.

2 Reach out with your left hand towards your toes as far as
you can. Hold for 30 seconds and repeat with the other leg.

Alternative stretch For an equally effective exercise that puts less
pressure on your lower back, sit on the edge of a bench and
place your right leg on the floor. Stretch the left leg along the
bench and extend your left hand to your toes while placing your
right hand on your knee. Hold this position for 30 seconds before
repeating with your other leg. This slow stretching pushes
muscles just beyond their usual range of movement.

Conditioning calves

The muscles that put a spring in your step and a leap in your stride should never be neglected when it comes to stretching.

REPS	1–2
TIME	30 secs

1 Place your feet on a step with the heel of your right foot overhanging the edge.

2 Slowly lower your right heel over the edge until you feel a slight tug in your lower leg. Hold that position for 30 seconds before repeating with the other foot.

Alternative stretch Stand about 1 metre (three feet) away from a wall and place your feet shoulder-width apart with your toes pointing forwards. Take a step forward with your left foot, letting the left knee bend, and place your hands flat against the wall, leaving your right foot flat on the floor. Now lean forward as far as you can without feeling discomfort. As you become more flexible increase your distance from the wall.

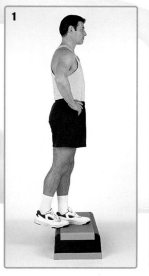

1

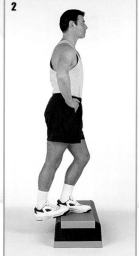

2

Back stretches

Make a special effort to stretch your lower back – it's been proved that fitter men experience less muscle strain in this area.

Spinal stretch

To hold the spine in place and allow complex body movements, the lower back is packed full of muscles, tendons, and ligaments. This makes it vulnerable to aches and strains, which means it's important to keep it as flexible as possible.

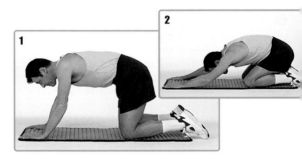

1 Get down on all fours positioning your hands directly beneath your shoulders. Make sure your head is pointed towards the ground.

2 Without moving your hands, sit back on your heels so that your arms are outstretched ahead of you. When doing this exercise take care not to let your back sag. By keeping it straight you won't put any undue stress on the spine.

Alternative stretch Get into the starting position described above and arch your back so that it's rounded towards the ceiling. Your posture should be something akin to a cat with its tail trapped in the door. Don't allow yourself to rock back on your heels. After this, let your back come down into the original position and repeat to loosen up the entire length of the spine.

Keep control

When doing any of these exercises, it's important not to overstretch your muscles. Use slow and controlled movements to push yourself until you feel a slight tug in the muscle. If you go any further than this you'll risk injury.

REPS 1–2
TIME 30 secs

1 Lie back with your arms stretched straight out at your sides and your palms facing the floor. While keeping the right leg extended, bend the left leg and put your left foot on the floor next to your right knee.

2 From this starting position twist your hips while keeping your upper body still. Turn your left knee over your right leg and push it downwards as far as it can go before it starts to feel uncomfortable. Try to prevent your left shoulder from lifting off the floor. By keeping it flat on the floor your upper back and shoulder will also benefit from the stretch. Hold the position and return to the start position before doing the same stretch on the other side.

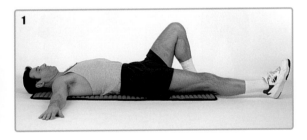

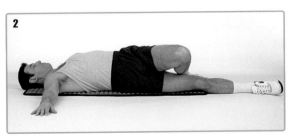

Side and chest stretches

These exercises will stretch muscles that determine the range of movement around the trunk and stop you getting chest soreness.

Avoid tugs or bounces

When doing this or any other stretch, don't be tempted to bounce when you reach for the stretch. If you push stretched muscles that bit further in short and quick bursts you risk tearing the muscle fibres. The effect is the same as overextending rubber bands.

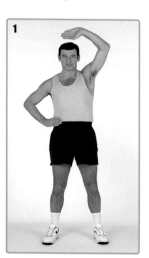

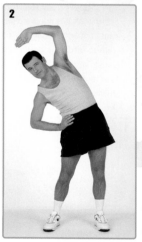

REPS **1–2**
TIME **30 SECS**

1 Stand up straight and bend your knees slightly with your feet should-width apart. Extend your left arm above your head and place your right hand on your hip, with the palm facing away from the body.

2 Bend sideways at the hip, reach your hand over your head, and move it to the right. Hold and repeat on the other side.

Pectoral stretch

There's no point having huge chest muscles if you can't flex them. This stretching exercise may not make your pectoral muscles (pecs) quiver like a professional body builder's, but it will stop you from getting sore across the chest after training. In all stretching exercises breathe normally. For some reason many of us hold our breath when we're holding a stretch. Slow, rhythmic breaths contribute to your stretch by helping you to relax. It's also the most efficient way of getting oxygen into your muscles.

REPS 1–2
TIME 30 SECS

1 Position yourself in a doorway or at the edge of a wall with your feet shoulder-width apart. Bend your elbow at 90° and place your hand and forearm against the wall. In this starting position your upper arm should be parallel with the floor and your forearm parallel with the wall.

2 Rotate your body slowly towards your right shoulder so that the raised left hand is drawn slightly behind your chest. Hold this position and repeat with your right arm.

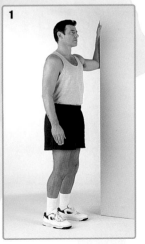

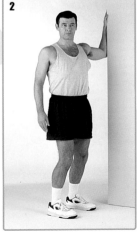

Index

Acknowledgements

The author would like to thank:
Wayne Campbell, Michelle Fitzmaurice, Michael Walsh,
Rachael Stock, and Jane Cooke.

Picture Credits

Octopus Publishing Group Ltd 21, 71, 76–77, 79, 80, 81, 103, 104,
112–113,/Steve Gorton 10–11, 23, 28, 28–29, 30–31, 38, 39, 40, 43,
49, 63, 70, 84, 127, 130 left, 131 right, 131 bottom right, 132–133,
136–137, 144, 146, 147 top, 147 centre, 147 bottom, 150–151, 154
left, 154 right, 154 b, 155 left, 155 right, 155 bottom left, 155 bottom
right, 158–159, 160–161, 161 top, 161 centre, 161 bottom, 162 top,
162 bottom, 162–163, 163 top, 163 centre, 163 bottom left, 163
bottom right, 164–165, 166 left,166 right, 167 left, 167 right, 167
bottom right, 168 left, 168 right, 169 left, 169 right, 170 left, 170
right, 170–171, 171 left, 171 right, 172 left, 172 right, 173 left, 173
right, 174 top, 174 bottom, 175 left, 175 right, 176 left, 176 right, 177
left, 177 right, 178 top, 178 bottom, 178–179, 179 left, 179 right, 180
left, 180 right, 180–181, 181 left, 181 right, 182 left, 182 right, 183
top, 183 bottom, 184 left, 184 right, 184–185, 185 left, 185
right,/Ruth Jenkinson 82–83,/James Johnson 14 bottom, 16, 17,
56,115,/Ray Moller 12–13, 14–15,/Steven Morris 26–27,/Roger Phillips
20,/Clive Streeter 15,/Halli Verrinder 37, 59, 63, 70, 98, 99, 101, 107,
107 bottom, 108, 111,/Paul Williams 4–5, 16–17, 20 centre bottom,
20 bottom; Rodale Images 2–3, 47, 138–139,/J P Hamel 1,
116–117,/Mitch Mandel 90–91; Science Photo Library/Tek Image
55,/Hattie Young 124–125; The Stock Market Photo Agency Inc 6, 9;
Tony Stone Images/Ziggy Kaluzny 122–123.